First published 1990 by Garland Publishing, Inc.

Published 2021 by Routledge
2 Park Square, Milton Park, Abingdon, Oxon OX14 4RN
605 Third Avenue, New York, NY 10017

Routledge is an imprint of the Taylor & Francis Group, an informa business

Library of Congress Cataloging-in-Publication Data

Derivan, William J., 1951–
Prevention education: a guide to research / William J. Derivan, Natalie Anne Silverstein.
p. cm. — (The Garland bibliographies in contemporary education; vol. 9) (Garland reference library of social science; vol. 524)
ISBN 0–8240–3716–2 (alk. paper)
1. Drug abuse—Prevention—Study and teaching (Secondary)—United States—Bibliography. 2. Alcoholism—Prevention—Study and teaching (Secondary)—United States—Bibliography. I. Silverstein, Natalie Anne, 1934– . II. Title. III. Series: Garland bibliographies in contemporary education; v. 9. IV. Series: Garland reference library of social science; v. 524.
Z7164.N17D44 1990
[HV5808]
016.36229'17—dc20 89–39996
CIP

ISBN 13: 978-0-8240-3716-1 (hbk)

CONTENTS

INTRODUCTION

PREVENTION EDUCATION

The problem of substance abuse has continued to escalate over the last 20 years, as is evidenced by all available prevalence data on substance abuse. These data demonstrate a continued need for research in the field of substance abuse and, specifically, in the field of prevention of substance abuse. Substance abuse has become a pervasive problem in our lives. It has escalated to where it touches all aspects of our society. Government leaders continue to identify substance abuse as one of our most significant problems and have given it the highest priority for our society's concern. The Governors of New York, New Jersey, and Connecticut have identified this as a shared concern in their State of the State addresses for 1988. President George Bush has indicated that he will continue to focus the attention of the Federal government on this problem. It has been noted that prior administrations have won some battles in the war against drugs, yet the war itself continues. It becomes our task as researchers and educators to join in this war, to develop educational programs and strategies to further this effort, to assist in enabling our youth to see a future without the need for, or reliance upon, substance abuse. This can best be done through the joint efforts of the education, mental health, and medical communities.

It is evident, through the continued and increased need for prevention services, that the objectives of prevention services have not fully been met. This is for a variety of reasons. One of these is a continued need for a research tool in the field of prevention education to determine and understand which programs have worked, why they have worked, and how to better the effects of these.

This volume focuses on education and offers a retrospective of the publications and research conducted in this field. This tool will be of assistance to teachers, administrators, supervisors, curriculum planners, and school boards, as well as psychologists, counselors, medical personnel, parents, youth agency workers, and others interested in prevention services and their development.

An important feature of this research tool is the commingling of the fields of education and prevention for the mutual goal of the enhancement of program development. "Enhancement" includes the tenets of the highest caliber of teaching, health care, and prevention services. It is through this commingling that prevention efforts will be established in the classroom.

Definitions

In order to provide a comprehensive base for work, we must first make the necessary distinctions between and among individuals and their degree of substance abuse. Let us clarify and build this base by explaining levels of prevention. We shall define prevention within the parameters of primary, secondary, and tertiary prevention. Primary prevention is defined as prevention of substance abuse with individuals who have never used drugs. Secondary prevention, as prevention of substance abuse with individuals who have experimented with chemicals and alcohol. These individuals are commonly referred to as "fence sitters." Finally, tertiary prevention is defined as prevention of continued substance abuse with individuals who are actively involved in using drugs. Tertiary prevention can also be viewed as treatment. This book will provide citations related to primary prevention: education prior to abuse; secondary prevention: education during early stages of abuse; and tertiary prevention: education during the later phases of abuse.

1.STRUCTURE OF BIBLIOGRAPHY

Topics Covered

This bibliography contains references to subjects from both primary and secondary sources, such as review of curriculum and curriculum guides, preservice and inservice teacher training manuals, reviews of formative and summative evaluations, evaluation guides from state and local projects, teacher training materials, articles from government documents, books, and monographs. Previously published bibliographies are included, as well as compilations and listings of materials and other resources. Also included are materials related to the identification of symptoms and signs of substance abuse. Equally important, and also included, are articles related to the effect of drug abuse on learning performance. Articles that relate to tertiary prevention strategies have been included due to the information they share related to the treatment process. These generally were services and treatment interventions designed for families. These articles and reviews are valuable in understanding the role the family plays in the etiology, prevention, and treatment of the substance abuse problem and will allow for a better understanding of essential concepts for incorporation into prevention efforts. Researchers will be interested in understanding the goals, objectives, and strategies of this type of prevention effort and may be helpful in developing the objectives that need to be met by primary and secondary levels of prevention efforts.

Other materials related to the development of special programs which meet the needs of learning disabled and handicapped students and their families identified as at risk and in need of primary, secondary, or tertiary prevention services have also been included.

Additionally, this guide contains a listing of periodicals and government publications available in this field. This guide is geared to furthering the endeavors of those who choose to continue developing services for those students identified as at risk. A research guide of this nature cannot be considered without providing its readers with further resources of related agencies, services, publications, and a listing of related support services for the families of these students. These are included in the Appendices. These resources will be helpful for those looking for additional information, access to services, technical assistance in program development, funding, etc.

Topics Not Covered

Our intention throughout the research phase of producing this book has been to focus towards inclusiveness rather than exclusiveness. Even with this objective, topics emerged that were unsuitable for a variety of reasons. We used as our criteria: relevancy of the topic; degree of usefulness for the reader; applicability to the research topic; and length of the proposed topic. It was felt that the excluded topics were better suited for future volumes.

Studies related to dissertations were generally excluded because they represented short term interventions of proposed treatments produced for academic studies. Few of these treatment programs presently exist, and there is the question as to whether these programs could be generalized to greater populations. Many dissertations have small population samples and cannot realistically be generalized to larger populations. In several cases, dissertations were included that were felt to have addressed populations large enough to be generalized to other populations or that were evaluations and studies of existing programs. The other dissertations that were included were considered valuable in that they presented unique ideas and or new insights into prevention theory and issues.

Topics and material related directly to the mental health field were excluded. We believe that these topics are too clinical in nature and target a specific audience. Again, we felt that materials for this special audience and these topics would be best covered in a separate volume. Articles which specifically related to the treatment process were excluded for reasons that are self-explanatory. This volume speaks to prevention and its relationship with education. The issue of treatment is an entirely separate field.

Through the process of research we encountered a great deal of literature published on the biomedical results of substance abuse. These generally were studies of the effects of specific drugs on learning performance, motor control and memory. Because of the confusing nature of these reports and the technical content they presented, there was concern as to whether this information would be suitable for the purposed audience and was, as such, excluded.

Sources of Reference

Extensive search methods were employed. Special data bases such as Drug Info/Alcohol and BRS were used. In addition, papers and articles were retrieved from DISC (Drug Information Service Center), HAZE (Hazelton Foundation), DIALOG, Educational Resources Information Center (ERIC), Current Index to Journals of Education (CIJE), Psychological Abstracts, Psychinfo, National Clearinghouse for Alcohol Information (NCALI), Social Science Abstracts, Educational Index, Resources in Education, Current Index to Journals in Education, and the world's literature in psychology and related disciplines in the behavioral sciences, as well as the resources of the National Institute on Alcoholism and Alcohol Abuse, the National Institute on Drug Abuse, the New York State Division of Substance Abuse, and the New York State Division of Alcoholism and Alcohol Abuse.

Types of Documents Included

Throughout the bibliography a variety of document types are listed. These include research reports, formative and summative evaluations, program descriptions, and program evaluations. They represent both journal articles, books, pamphlets, published curricula, curriculum guides, and other published works. In addition, government publications on the topic were retrieved and included, some reviews of audio-visual materials were included. Listings and previously published bibliographies were also included.

Some of the documents listed in the bibliography are reviews of other research. These were found to be valuable due to the idea of replicating programs, validating other prevention attempts, and other information that they make available. It was felt important that articles included have a broad base of interest for readers and the ability to stimulate further research.

2. HISTORY OF PREVENTION EDUCATION

In reviewing the trends in prevention techniques, ideas and recommendations for future research become clear. The earliest prevention programs were, essentially, scare tactics that hoped to scare students into not using drugs. Evaluations of these types of prevention efforts indicate that these were unsuccessful. In some evaluations it is noted that this type of prevention effort may have, in fact, stimulated an interest in students experimenting with substances and consequently, initiated substance abuse, thereby, causing what it had initially attempted to prevent.

More recent attempts at prevention have learned from these earlier experiences and have developed more social models whereby developmental issues are incorporated into the prevention curriculum. These programs generally build on issues of communication, self-esteem, the ability to defend against negative peer pressure, etc. It appears that these programs are having much more success in the prevention of substance abuse. The programs having the best success are those that have blended a variety of different professional disciplines as well as incorporating the families of students into prevention efforts, allowing for a more holistic approach to prevention to be developed.

Regardless of the approach to prevention, what becomes clear is that a great deal more work has to be done. Prevention education has to be initiated in the classroom, specifically in the early grades, and followed in all other aspects of a student's life which include community, family, and social spheres.

3. A GUIDE TO USING THIS BIBLIOGRAPHY

The reader may access information in this book by using the subject, title, or author index. Although several authors names appear again and again, the subject index will be useful for most people. The subject index is expansive and provides reference sources for all materials and subject topics referred to in the articles cited. Another interesting feature of the bibliography is references related to periodicals about drugs and alcohol abuse. The appendices list additional sources of information that include resources for technical assistance, support services, program development resources, periodicals that may not have appeared in the text of the bibliography, government agencies developed for assistance in program development, funding, etc.

Many entries have applicability to more than one section. These entries will have been cross referenced to more than one section. This is noted through the use of an asterisk rather than an entry number. The cross referenced entry will refer you to the primary entry where you will find the narrative description of the entry. No entry has more than one entry number.

4. OVERVIEW OF BIBLIOGRAPHIC TOPICS

The bibliographic entries are divided and entered in seven main categories with some categories having sub-listings: (1) Prevention Programs-School Based; (a) School Based, (b) Teacher Training, (c) School Administrators' Guides; (2) Youth and Prevention; (a) Program Development, (b) Program Evaluations and Reviews; (c) Peer Pressure; (3) Curricula/Materials; (4) Learning Performance; (5) Prevention; (a) Community Based, (b) Multi-Stage Models; (6) Family Systems; (a) Family Effects on Prevention, (b) Therapeutic Interventions, (c) Role of Parents; (7) Publications. Following the bibliographic entries are the Appendices that present other sources of information, services, and publications. All material is incorporated into the author, subject, and title indexes.

I. Prevention-School Based

Studies of prevention programs are included under this title. Specific attention was placed initially on programs that could be replicated in other schools and school programs. These categories eventually developed into three categories; School Based, Teacher Training, School Administrators' Guides. It was felt that the three categories should remain under the larger heading as they are all related to the provision of prevention services in school-based approaches. In addition, all three categories are related to school personnel at the variety of levels that are represented in the school. The section on school programs speaks directly to programs that have been developed in schools and that may have applicability to other school systems. The second section, Teacher Training, offers examples of Teacher Training curricula, evaluations of training attempts, and gives considerations for the development of other Teacher Training projects to increase staff skills in prevention issues. This section will be useful for anyone who wishes to develop inservice and preservice training models for staff to initially develop skills in teaching staff that will allow for prevention efforts to begin in the classroom, as well as in the overall school system. The last section, School Administrators' Guides, offers research on the development of policy and programs for consideration by school administrators, school board members, and other administrative bodies.

II. Youth and Prevention

Articles under this heading present material for the development of prevention programs as well as the evaluation of previously developed programs and are presented in three sections; Program Development, Program Evaluation and Reviews, and Peer Pressure. Evaluations and reviews of other research on prevention will also be found in these sections.

The first section, Program Development, presents programs that span a variety of methods used in prevention. These all relate to the education of students against the use of substances through cognitive development and enhancement of self. The second section, Program Evaluations and Reviews, includes formative and summative program evaluations as well as evaluations of community and school attempts in responding to the drug and alcohol abuse of their particular area. These articles will be of interest to those also interested in the development of programs. Reviews of many programs were included in this section that were offered as both school and community based.

The third section of this chapter, Peer Pressure, examines the role that it plays in the etiology and prevention of substance abuse. It is widely accepted that most substance abuse is the result of negative peer pressure in conjunction with other variables. This section outlines and describes programs than enable students to defend themselves against negative peer pressure, discusses the role of peer pressure on the development of substance abuse, discusses methods and means for teaching staff to develop self-esteem within students to make them less susceptible to negative peer pressure, and describes programs for the development of positive peer pressure for the prevention of substance abuse problems. These articles describe developing positive peer pressure within a school for the prevention of substance abuse, as well as co-opting students into school-wide campaigns against drugs.

III. Curricula/Materials

Articles, books, and references presented in this category all represent attempts, through curricula, to develop an ability in students not to use substances. Many innovative means of instruction are included. Curricula for all grade levels are included, as well as curricula for a variety of minority groups, exceptional education students, bilingual instruction, and cultural means of addressing curriculum. Many of the articles cited in this section present materials that are available for teaching staff to further the prevention efforts within their class. Resource guides for further investigation, as well as curriculum development resources are included.

IV. Learning Performance

The effects of drugs and alcohol on the ability of a student to learn and to retain facts is of interest to all teachers and educators. There has been a limited amount of research done in this area. The majority of research done in this area is laboratory research conducted as biochemical studies with the use of laboratory animals. These articles were viewed as inappropriate for the target audience and not included. What was included were studies of students where the effects of substance abuse on task and memory recall were measured and reported in a fashion that was less technical and, hence, more useful to researchers. This section of our research is the subject that has received the least amount of attention of past researchers.

V. Prevention

Program descriptions that targeted youth, directly and indirectly, were included under this category. Two sections are included: Community Based, and Multi-stage Models. The first section, Community Based, describes programs that were generally offered through community efforts as adjuncts to educational programs, not as primary parts of the educational institution. It was felt that these were important to include in that many of these programs were viewed as part of after-school activities or programs school administrators would be interested seeing developed as part of extra-curricula programs. Many of these programs require the assistance of parent groups, community groups, as well as the school community. Research indicates that services jointly developed by schools, communities, and parents have much better success in preventing substance abuse than those developed as individual efforts.

VI. Family Systems

All students exist as part of family systems. Therefore, a research guide on prevention for educators would not be complete without discussing the effects families have on the development and prevention of substance abuse in students. Much of what the teacher sees in the classroom is behavior that has been learned at home with the family of origin. To fully understand this behavior it is important to first have an understanding of the family process. Articles included in this section describe the effects that families have on the use of substances and prevention efforts, articles on therapeutic interventions and programs that involve families, as well as the role parents play in both prevention and treatment. Some articles represent tertiary prevention attempts. These were included due to their applicability to pure prevention efforts and due to the insight they offer into the overall family process as well as allowing for a better understanding of what prevention programs should be targeted towards. It was also felt desirable for researchers to become aware of the multidimensional role of the entire family process and its effect on students, their abusing behaviors, and subsequently on the prevention of substance abuse.

VIII. Publications

Articles that had relevance to the primary topic of Prevention Education, yet did not directly fall under any of the above mentioned categories, were included in this section. These included many government publications, previously published bibliographies, listings, resource guides, and other general articles.

Appendices

It has been mentioned that a volume of this type would not be complete without a listing of further resources for researchers. These are included in the two appendices. The first appendix provides researchers with a listing of agencies, services, and programs developed for the purposes of providing technical assistance, referrals, materials, funding, and information for individuals interested in the areas of drug and alcohol abuse and prevention. The second appendix provides a listing of periodicals and journals that had not previously been mentioned in the bibliography but that offer articles and information on the subject of substance abuse and prevention.

5. FUTURE DIRECTIONS OF RESEARCH

The earliest attempts at prevention of substance abuse are described as scare tactics offered to deter students from wanting to experiment with substances. Although offered in good conscience, these attempts actually had a reverse effect and stimulated an interest to experiment with substances. Recent attempts now use a more multidimensional approach to develop social and internal mechanisms in students to guard against the social forces that lead students to use substances. It could be inferred from the constant increase in the need for treatment services and the requests for prevention services that much more has to be learned about substance abuse and prevention efforts, what programs work and what ones do not.

The majority of research published and available on prevention education has been conducted as individual attempts at prevention. Many of these publications offer little or no empirical evidence to support the efforts at prevention. The articles do give future researchers a basis to build from, in that the program designs outlined will be helpful to those interested in replication of these efforts, although future efforts must include clearer evaluation processes to ensure the success or failure of these projects. Only then will we begin to understand the underlying processes of successful prevention efforts. No tool exists for the purpose of evaluating either the programmatic or individual effects of prevention services.

Several issues come to mind when thinking what directions should be taken in future prevention efforts. It is clear that prevention efforts, in addition to substance abuse, must take a more holistic approach and encompass alcohol, suicide, health issues, and other social concerns that have an impact on youth.

Areas that have not been investigated but that certainly warrant further study include prevention efforts based on the traditions and concepts of Alcoholics Anonymous and Narcotics Anonymous. These programs are built on the concepts of a self-help fellowship of recovering people that offer support and assistance to each other. These programs have demonstrated an incredible amount of success in the treatment of both alcohol and drug abuse.

In conclusion, we would like to affirm our commitment and belief in the role education can play in the prevention of drug and alcohol abuse, as well as other forms of destructive behaviors. Our intention in preparing this work has been to stimulate an interest in research in the development of viable programs and research that will better meet the needs of students. It is our hope that this bibliography will form a base from which future research can develop.

W.J.D.
2/89

Prevention Education

PREVENTION PROGRAMS

School Based Programs

1. Anderson, D.S., & Gadaleto, A.F. (1976). That happy feeling--An innovative model for a campus alcohol education program. Ratford, VA: Ratford University.

   Tells the reader how to establish a positive education program on campus. There are numerous examples, photos, pamphlets, questionnaires, and a complete how-to guide. A desirable tool for all campus groups, whether for an organized alcohol education effort or a group of concerned teachers and students.

2. California State Department of Education. (1979). Better schools, better people: Schools can help to prevent drug and alcohol abuse. Sacramento, CA: Author.

   Presents documentation on 25 school-based drug abuse prevention activities and experiences. Projects are described in terms of their design, implementation, and assessment components as well as the roles played by various school personnel, community agencies, school superintendents and other key personnel. Contains lists of contacts, printed materials, clearinghouse, and training resources.

3. Carlisle Area School District. (1970). A program for the prevention of drug abuse: Kindergarten-Adult. Carlisle, PA: Author.

   Attempts to identify the school's responsibility and program with regard to drug education and the prevention of drug abuse among young people. The introduction provides a sample policy statement on drug education and lists seven areas of program responsibility the school should undertake.

4. Cohen, S. (1976). Drug use, misuse, and abuse incidents among elementary school children. Journal of drug education, 6(3), 247-251.

   Describes the trend towards younger grade level children abusing drugs and emphasizes that the drug problem in America continues to spread rapidly.

5. Dembo, R. and others. (1976). Drug abuse prevention: The awareness, experience, and opinions of junior and senior high school students in New York State. Report No. 2 of Winter 1974-75 Survey. New York: New York State Office of Drug Abuse Services.

   Assesses student attitude toward, awareness of, and figures on current use of drugs in New York State junior and senior high schools. It also attempts to define programs and services youths feel are most appropriate and desirable. It represents the issues from the point of view of the youth being serviced.

6. Frank, P. (1974, April). An effective approach to drug education. Paper presented at the Annual Meeting of the American Educational Research Association, Chicago, IL.

   Discusses the notion that traditional methods of drug abuse prevention, i.e. scare tactics, do not work. The author suggests that schools direct their attention toward helping the child develop a good self-concept and teaching decision making skills. Descriptions of the You and Your Decision Project are given. In this project, written, audio visual, and workshop materials were developed to help parents and teachers create an environment in which a child can learn about the decision-making process.

7. Galant, R., and Moncrieff, N. (1974). Counseling for drug abuse. Searchlight: Relevant resources in high interest areas. Ann Arbor, MI: ERIC Clearinghouse on Counseling and Personnel Services.

Describes 81 document abstracts that refer to drug and alcohol abuse, prevention, and prevention education programs.

8. Grabb, J. (1981). Of mice and myths. Grassroots, 17(9/81).

Presents a program developed by the Texas Commission on Alcoholism called SMILE, Student Myth-Information and Learning Experiences. It uses realistic examples and projects to heighten student awareness to the real life consequences of alcohol abuse.

9. Haun, D. (1975). Where kids teach kids. Teacher, 92(7), 59-61.

Describes a program that uses peer teaching as a means of raising self-esteem, which is described as a causative factor in substance abuse.

* Hewitt, L. (1982). Current status of alcohol education programs for youth. In: Alcohol and health mono. No. 4: Special populations. Washington, DC: U.S. Government Printing Office.

See No. 102.

* Kopita, R. (1973). Searchlight: Relevant resources in high interest areas. 4U update search. Counseling for drug abuse. Ann Arbor, MI: ERIC Clearinghouse on Counseling and Personnel Services.

See No. 596.

10. Kriner, R., and others. (1973). Educational approaches to the prevention of non-therapeutic use of drugs. Alexandria, VA: Human Resources Research Organization.

Presents the results of a four-phase effort in which guidelines describing the qualities and characteristics of a successful drug education program were formulated.

11. Kruger, W.S. (1972). Education for parenthood and the schools. Washington, DC: Bureau of Elementary And Secondary Education.

Describes the school-related programs of the Education for Parenthood Project. The purpose is to provide knowledge and skills to enable parents to be more effective.

* Lopez, T. and Starkey, K. (1976). A primary prevention drug education program for school children: An attempt at evaluation. Paper presented at the Annual Meeting of the American Educational Research Association, San Francisco, CA.

See No. 271.

12. Myers, E. (1973). Applying a casual approach to drug education. Journal of drug education, 3 (4), 415-418.

Describes a preventive drug education program developed for grades K-12. The core of this program is developed around education in human behavior.

13. National Institute on Alcohol Abuse and Alcoholism. (1984). Prevention plus: Involving schools, parents, and the community in alcohol and drug education. Rockville, MD: Author.

Presents materials and gives outlines for teacher training, curricula, model programs for schools, model policies developed for schools, parent education programs, guidelines for school personnel, community approaches, early intervention strategies, risk reduction programs, and prevention ideas. Further, the authors suggest ways that communities, parents, and schools can better work together in developing prevention efforts.

14. Operation Uplift...(1975). <u>NJEA review, 49</u> (3), 34.

Describes a model policy on student care and counseling for prevention of drug and alcohol dependency. It was adopted by the Department of School Nurses through funding by the National Educational Association for Operation Uplift--Better Health for Better Learning.

15. Pascale, P. and Streit, F. (1974, April). <u>A model for drug prevention in the schools--Critical Period of Intervention</u>. Paper presented at the 59th Annual Meeting of the American Educational Research Association, Chicago, IL.

Describes the Critical Period of Intervention (CPI), a model prevention program designed for schools, unique in that its underlying theories are based on the psychological principles of stage development and critical period theories. The program consists of four phases: identification, diagnosis, intervention, and evaluation. The author notes that this design allows for identification of high risk students as well as for intervention of students that are experimenting with drugs.

16. Pollack, B. (1972). Decision-Making--A key to prevention of drug abuse. <u>Journal of drug education,2</u>(4), 383-389.

Describes the role and the importance of decision-making in schools as a vehicle for drug abuse prevention. Decision-making is examined as a process that may be structured to make learning meaningful and give youngsters the skills and resources necessary to face up to social pressures involved in the spread of drug abuse.

17. Resnik, H. (1978). <u>It starts with people: Experiences in drug abuse prevention</u>. Rockville, MD: National Institute on Drug Abuse.

Describes several different approaches to prevention education and addresses a variety of disciplines and professions. It draws on the experiences of several dozen drug abuse prevention programs that were visited and assessed as part of an intensive research and review process. Strategies and educational techniques for prevention programs are emphasized.

18. Room, R. (1972). Strategies of prevention and alcohol opinion campaigns. <u>Journal of alcohol and drug education, 18</u>(1), 6-8.

    Discusses the role of definitions in the establishment of prevention efforts. The author contends that using a definition that allows for a distinction between normal drinking and alcoholic drinking is a step in the wrong direction.

19. Ryan, W. (1976). Project youth: An approach to drug abuse. <u>Guidance and counseling, 10</u> (4), 270-278.

    Describes a drug prevention program for preadolescent children. The program is designed to effect and develop self-esteem and a positive self-concept through the use of small group work and positive peer influence. A program evaluation shows that it is influential in changing student characteristics.

20. Sheppard, M.A. (1976). <u>Barriers to the implementation of a new school based alcohol education program</u>. Toronto, Canada: Addiction Research Foundation.

    Describes an alcohol education program offered to school boards in the Canadian Province of Toronto. Difficulties with implementation of this project as well as recommendations for other programs are made.

21. Shields, E. and others. (1973, March). <u>Choicepoint: A peer group model for facilitating decision making</u>. Paper presented at the American College Personnel Association, Atlanta, GA.

Presents a peer led decision-making facilitation group for college level students. The authors assert that decison making appears to be a major factor in maladaptive behavior, and that prevention of problems may occur through responsible decisions and behavior.

22. Smith, K. (1983). Alcohol and other drug abuse prevention and intervention: A pilot project for high school. Paper presented at the conference titled Working with Adolescent Alcohol/Drug Problems: Assessment, Intervention, and Treatment. Madison, WI.

Describes a program where clinical staff worked with educational personnel to develop programs within educational environments. The project has a dual focus: the first being to train and educate staff and students; the second was to develop and implement policies and procedures. Project goals included increasing student and staff awareness of specific prevention and intervention program strategies and evaluating the impact of the programs.

23. Stolz, P. and Van Der Heide, G. (1983, May). School/community intervention workshop: A workshop on the CADAP (Community Alcohol and Drug Abuse Prevention). Paper presented at the National Drug Institute, Brisbane, Australia.

Presents a report on a community workshop designed to develop an understanding of the Community Alcohol and Drug Abuse Prevention Project. Outlines the philosophy and approach to prevention issues used by the CADAP group.

* Swisher, J. and Horman, R. (1970). Drug abuse prevention. Journal of college student personnel, 2(5), 337-340

See No. 347.

Teacher Training

24. Abrams, I. and Hawkins, B. (1962). Information about narcotics--Resource material for teachers. Chicago, IL: Chicago Board of Education.

Presents a short history of substance abuse with an explanation of addiction and methods of its prevention. Includes ways in which teachers may identify students who are abusing drugs. Much of the material presented is dated and relates solely to physical addiction and disregards the social aspects of drug abuse prevention.

* American Association for Health, Physical Education, and Recreation. (1969). Research book for drug abuse information. Washington, DC: National Science Teachers Association.

See No. 586.

25. Campbell, J. and Swanchak, J. (1981, March). Essential elements for the in-service training of teachers in drug abuse prevention. Paper presented at the Annual Meeting of the Eastern Educational Research Association, Philadelphia, PA.

Describes the efforts and what influences these efforts in regards to drug abuse prevention programs and their development in schools. It describes the key person as the classroom teacher. Research is cited where teacher attitudes, skills and abilities were measured. These findings clearly indicated that teachers that were empathic towards prevention and trained properly enabled programs to succeed more readily. The author calls for more formal training to be offered to teachers.

* Center for Alcohol Studies. (1980). Recent topics in alcohol studies. Piscataway, NJ: Rutgers University.

See No. 589.

26. Cohen, S. (1977). Behavioral objectives for the drug education preparation of K-3 elementary school teachers. Journal of drug education, 7(1), 1-14.

Describes a study and a proposed program for the training of K-3 elementary school teachers. Considerations for future studies are made.

* Conroy, G. and Brayer, H. (1978). Teen involvement for drug abuse prevention. Administrators guide. (Report No. DHEW-ADM-78-624). Rockville, MD: National Institute of Drug Abuse.

See No. 72

27. Cowan, J.S. (1980). About alcohol education, Perspectives for educators. Grassroots,1 (1/81).

Presents a partial explanation for the failure of alcohol prevention programs and makes suggestions for better perfecting these services. Suggestions included materials related to teaching students decision making skills.

28. DiCicco, L., et al. (1983). Teacher training in alcohol education: Changes over three years. Journal of alcohol and drug education, 29 (1), 12-26.

Reports the findings of pre and post tests given to teachers that participated in a CASPAR alcohol education workshop. Results indicate that a substantial increase in knowledge about alcoholism and alcohol was achieved, that there was some change in general attitude toward drinking, and a greater perception that teenagers are potential alcohol abusers. These were maintained at two and three year follow-ups and teachers reported using CASPAR curriculum material in instruction.

29. Eiseman, S., Robinson, J., and Zapata, V. (1984). M.D.A.: A multi-disciplinary approach for teacher effectiveness training in drug education. Journal of drug education, 14(4), 357-367.

Describes a teacher training model using a multi-disciplinary approach that included the principles of psychology, sociology, health science, communications, and legal aspects of substance abuse. Topics to be covered include responsibility for drug education, theories and models of drug abuse, community action programs, and research findings.

30. Floyd, J., Lang, R., and Lotsoff, A. (1975). Drug education: Suggested guidelines for conducting an effective course for teachers. Journal of the American College Health Association, 24(1), 15-19.

Describes the concepts of a pre-service or in-service training program for teachers in the area of drug education. Drug abuse is viewed as a symptom of basic human needs unfulfilled by other means so that the goal of drug education must be to encourage a better way of gaining satisfaction and solving problems.

31. Frederick, C. (1976). Trends in mental health: Self destructive behavior among younger age groups. (Report Number DHEW-ADM-76-365). Rockville, MD: National Institute on Drug Abuse.

Discusses methods of recognizing and responding to behavior that can culminate in suicide, with emphasis on adolescents and young adults. Incidence and types of behavior are described and include drug abusing behaviors, clues to aid in the identification of potential suicides are provided, and ten preventive steps are recommended.

32. Griffin, T. and Svendsen, R. (1980). Student Assistance Program: How it works. Center City, MN: Hazeldon Foundation.

    Describes a complete student assistance program that offers services to students that are troubled by physical, emotional, social, legal, sexual, medical, family, or chemical abuse problems while improving the quality of education in school. Unique to this program is that it is developed to use existing personnel rather than develop new staff positions and focuses on educational issues rather than reshifting the focus to social problems. Useful as a guide for developing in-service workshops for educational staff.

33. Gidden, N. and Rollin, S. (1975). A didactic-experiential model for an in-service workshop on drug abuse education. Journal of drug education, 5(4), 359-370.

    Describes a one day workshop on program development for drug education. It combines didactic features with group techniques to generate a practical list of needs, resources, and programs for use in public schools.

34. Handbook for the prevention and control of drug problems. (1970). Parsippany, NJ: Troy Hills Department of Education.

    Presents guidelines for teachers relative to drug abuse. Suggests steps necessary to follow in attempting to prevent and/or guide students with a drug problem. Stress is placed on helping each student, individually, to understand the forces affecting him or her, and in helping him or her form the necessary attitudes to cope with each individual cause which may lead to drug-abusing behavior.

35. Harper, F. (1975). Alcohol education: The role of the teacher. Phi delta kappan, 57(4), 259.

Suggests that the teacher's role should emphasize prevention rather than remediation of alcohol abuse and provides sources of instructional meterials on alcohol and places of help for parents and students with alcohol-related problems.

36. Hochhauser, M. (1981). Ethical issues in academic substance abuse consultation. Paper presented at the 89th Annual Convention of the American Psychological Association, Los Angeles, CA.

Presents two important ethical issues in the field of consultation for substance abuse. These are the abuse of the role of a consultant and the fact that many drug education prevention programs actually increase drug-using behaviors. Suggestions are given for how the psychological consultant can attempt to improve the methodological quality of substance abuse programs, while simultaneously ensuring that ethical standards are maintained.

37. Horan, J. and others. (1973). A training model for drug abuse prevention: Content and evaluation. Journal of drug education, 3 (2), 121-126.

Describes the content and evaluation of a training center for drug abuse prevention. Through a series of four workshops, teams of students, educators, and community leaders received intensive training in behavioral group counseling focused on alternatives to drug use. Evaluation using several criteria indicated that the goals of the training center were successfully achieved.

38. Juel, C. (1981). A process and outcome evaluation of an effective in-service training program for junior high school teachers: Second year results. Napa, CA: Pacific Institute for Research and Evaluation.

Describes a training program for teachers of junior high school in which the focus of the training was effective classroom management. Teachers were taught techniques in discipline, communication, and self-esteem enhancement. The goal of the in-service training was to make teachers more responsive to affective and cognitive needs of students.

39. Ketterman, C. (1969). A drug abuse workshop. School counselor, 17(2), 99-100.

Briefly describes a program for high school personnel to increase awareness and acquire a realistic viewpoint from which to assist the user or potential user. Includes addresses for source materials.

40. Link, W. and others. (1977). Facts about drug abuse: Trainers' manual. Gaitersburg, MD: National Drug Abuse Center for Training and Resource Development.

Presents a modular drug abuse trainers' manual containing all course-specific materials. Contains the course goals and objectives, time and activity sheets, trainer guidelines, process notes, exercise instructions, detailed lectures, and supplementary information.

41. Link, W. and others. (1979). Drugs in perspective: Trainers' manual and resource guide. Gaitersburg, MD: National Drug Abuse Center for Training and Resources Development.

Presents a manual to be used in the training of those helping professionals working with youth, overseas military personnel, and community service organizations in drug abuse prevention and treatment. All materials, lecture outlines, and other relevant materials are included.

42. May, F. and McDougall, P. (1967). Developing assessment instruments for measuring the effects of group counseling in the Teacher Education Program At Washington State Univer-

sity, Final Report. Pullman, WA: Washington State University.

Reports of the findings of the Washington University study for the evaluation of group counseling sessions designed to enhance the mental health of prospective elementary school teachers.

43. Mayer, V. (1982). Health education for prospective teachers: Is it effective? Journal of school health, 52 (8), 491-494.

Reports on the findings of pre and post tests after completion of an undergraduate course in health education and drug abuse. Students indicated that they felt more confident in their ability to recognize and deliver first aid in the classroom as well as in their ability to teach health education, and that it increased their interest to teach health education.

44. Michigan State Dept. of Education. (1975). Substance Abuse Prevention Education Program. Evaluation Report, 1974-1975. Lansing, MI: Author.

Describes a program that was developed to have an effect on the youth of the schools, parents of the students; covers the nature of substance abuse, its causes and effects.

45. Miezitis, S. and Orme, M. (1977). Innovation in school psychology. Toronto, Canada: Author.

Presents several issues for the school psychologist that relate to drug abuse identification and training. Among the topics indicated are in-service training, issues in drug abuse counseling, and a consultation model.

46. Moskowitz, J. and others. (1981). The effects of classroom management teacher training primary prevention program on fifth-grade students. Napa, CA: Pacific Institute for Research and Evaluation.

Describes the teacher training program named Effective Classroom Management II-Elementary. Highlights techniques in communication, classroom management, and self-esteem enhancement. The goals are to make classroom environments more responsive to students' affective and cognitive needs, thereby fostering positive attitudes, behaviors, and norms regarding self, peers, and school.

47. National Drug Abuse Prevention Program. (1970). Compact,4 (3), 25.

Describes a prevention program that is geared to develop in teaching staff skills to identify and respond appropriately to substance abuse problems.

* National Institute on Drug Abuse. (1980). Angel dust in four American cities: An ethnographic study of PCP users. Kensington, MD: Author.

See No. 602.

48. National Institute of Education. (1977). Humanizing preservice teacher education: Strategies for alcohol and drug abuse prevention. Washington, DC: Author.

Presents reports of six demonstration projects and one research project engaged in primary prevention of alcohol and drug abuse prevention. The programs focused very little on actual drug and alcohol abuse but attempted to deal with causes rather than symptoms. The goal of these projects was to find ways to humanize teacher education and to develop teachers who would create humanistic environments in the schools to offset student need to seek external gratification through drug abuse.

49. New York State, Division of Alcoholism and Alcohol Abuse. (1979). Fetal alcohol syndrome. New York: Author.

Includes brochures, posters, the task-force

report, sample teaching kit, buttons, and local coordinators' manual. The manual and teaching kit are designed for copying by schools and organizations. Extremely useful at all levels of teacher training research. Presents detailed information on the life-long effects and consequences of alcohol on the unborn fetus.

50. New York State Education Department. (1978). Annotated resource guide for alcohol, tobacco, and other drug abuse/misuse prevention education programs. Elementary level. Albany, NY: Author.

Provides teachers with a selective list of instructional aids and resources for use in drug education programs. It provides some guidance in choosing, from the items listed, those to use at the local level.

51. Nortoft, B. and Dorn, N. (1982). Health careers: Teachers manual. London, England: Institute for the Study of Drug Dependence.

Describes curriculum and teacher training activities that enable students to develop the ability to make healthy decisions in regard to drug abuse.

* Nowlis, H. (1977). Statement before the Subcommittee on Alcoholism and Drug Abuse, Committee on Human Resources, United States Senate. Washington, DC: United States Government Printing Office.

See No. 609.

* Nowlis, H. (1980, March). Prevention is not easy. Paper presented at the First Pan-Pacific Conference on Drugs and Alcohol, Canberra, Australia.

See No. 610.

52. Pacificon Productions. (1980). Saying no: Drug abuse prevention ideas for the classroom. Rockville, MD: National Institute on Drug Abuse.

Designed to provide drug abuse prevention ideas for the junior school teacher. The information, activities and resources address the educational portion of the prevention continuum defined by the National Institute on Drug Abuse. Includes research findings that will help the teacher, specific prevention activities to be incorporated into existing curriculum, and a list of resources for additional information and ideas about prevention and the role of the classroom teacher.

* Polzella, S. and Selinger, M. (1981). Teacher intervention for the adolescent substance abuser. Arlington, VA: Educational Document Reproduction Service.

See No. 39.

53. Reagen, M. (Ed.). (1971). Readings for the Institute for Drug Education at Syracuse. Syracuse, NY: Continuing Education Center for the Public Service.

Intended primarily for teachers, this book of 17 readings is an attempt to provide a brief, descriptive overview of some of the complexities of the drug abuse problem.

54. Ramsey, G. and Barnes, L. (1976, May). Drugs, society and personal choice: A summer school for teachers. Paper presented at the Annual Convention of the Canadian Guidance and Counseling Association, Halifax, Nova Scotia.

Presents a course outline for teachers to develop skills in drug abuse prevention, and the ability to assist students in skill building in decision making. The development, planning and implementation of this program are presented.

* Rehrer, R. (1982). Now what do I do? A guide on alcohol and drugs for youth. St. Louis, MO: Concordia Publishing House.

See No. 399.

55. Resnikoff, A. and others. (1976). Training counselors and teachers in behavioral contracting: Three years of outcomes. Presented as a collection of papers at the annual meeting of the American Education Research Association, San Francisco, CA.

Describes a program used to upgrade the skills of teachers as they relate to drug abuse, alcohol abuse, and other relevant mental health issues. Although the papers are varied in content, specific attention is placed on the role of the teacher as it relates to drug and alcohol abuse prevention through classroom interactions.

56. Rogers, D. (1977). An inventory of educational improvement efforts in the New York City Public Schools. New York, NY: Educational Planning Foundation.

Describes the various programs developed and implemented by the N.Y.C.-Board of Education since 1970 until the publication date. Describes various programs that include educational programs, programs for traditional and alternative settings, public sector programs, private sector programs, vocational and prevocational programs, bi-lingual programs, programs for the handicapped, drug prevention programs, etc. It further describes the staff and financial resources needed to develop such programs.

57. Safford, P., Deighan, W., Corder,L. and Miller, W. (1975). Training teachers for drug abuse prevention: A humanistic approach. Journal of drug education, 5 (4), 335-349.

Describes a staff development model that sought to bring about the personal involvement of both teachers and students. Drug use is defined within the context of personal needs, values, and decision making, implying the need for a personalized and affectively oriented approach. The authors suggest that program goals are being met.

58. Sherman, R., Lojkuitz, S. and Steckiewicz, N. (1979). The ADE Program: An approach to the realities of alcohol and drug education. Chicago, IL: Chicago Department of Health.

Describes a teacher training program provided for the teachers of the Chicago Public School System. It is designed to equip teachers with the ability to initiate alcohol and drug abuse educational activities.

59. Sherman, R., Lojkuitz, S. and Rusch, L. (1984). An evaluation of the ADE program: A teacher training strategy in alcohol and drug education. Journal of alcohol and drug education, 30 (1), 66-76.

Reports pre and post data from 92 teachers that participated in the Alcohol and Drug Education (ADE) teacher training program. Results indicate that the program led to significant improvement in assertiveness and in knowledge and attitudes concerning drug and alcohol abuse.

* Shields, E. and others. (1973, March). Choicepoint: A peer group model for facilitating decision making. Paper presented at the American College Personnel Association, Atlanta, GA.

See No. 21.

60. Shute, R. and Swisher, J. (1974). Training models for drug abuse prevention: Recommendations for the future. Journal of drug education, 4 (2), 169-178.

Describes and provides examples of the three major training modalities currently in vogue. The strengths and weaknesses of each are examined and then integrated to build a recommended model for future training efforts.

* Sieber, J. and others. (1976). The effects of learning when to be uncertain on children's knowledge and use of drugs. R and D Memorandum No. 144. Stanford, CA: Stanford University, Center for Research and Development in Teaching.

See No. 333.

61. Silverstein, S. (Ed.), and others. (1971). Experiments in mental health training: Project summaries. Bethesda, MD: National Institute of Mental Health.

Reports on summaries of mental health training projects conducted under grants from the National Institute of Mental Health. These programs were developed to address the training needs of a variety of staff with different educational backgrounds. Materials and course outlines are provided.

62. Simon, R. (Ed.), and others. (1975). Explorations in mental health training: Project summaries. Rockville, MD: National Institute of Mental Health.

Describes 176 pilot projects that were developed for the training of mental health personnel. These programs were developed with an eye towards staff with a variety of educational backgrounds. A description of materials and course outlines are provided.

* Swanson, J. (1978). The "No Win": Drug education evaluation problems. Journal of drug education,8 (2), 125-129.

See No. 344.

63. Systems Management Corp. (1982). Source book: December 1982-1983. Miami, FL: Author.

Provides access to information in all aspects of training. Describes courses developed at government expense as well as the organizations that have the capacities to deliver these. Thirty-five courses are described that address the areas of alcohol abuse, drug abuse, and prevention issues.

64. Tate, C. (1970). In-service education for teachers. Science teacher, 37(6), 49-50.

Describes the basic philosophy, programs, and areas of concern in a teacher education program on drug abuse and concludes that drug education programs should emphasize the drug user and social matrix instead of the chemicals, include all levels of school personnel, as well as involve and focus on the entire community.

65. Texas Education Agency, Austin Division of Crime Prevention and Drug Education. (1975). A Framework for crime prevention and drug education in Texas: Desirable teacher competencies. Austin, TX: Author.

Provides guidelines for both teachers and students for their program of crime prevention and drug education. It describes the necessary teacher competencies in skills and attitudes in the secondary schools.

* U.S. Department of Health and Human Services. (1980). Beyond the three R's: Training teachers for effective education. Rockville, MD: Author.

See No. 357.

* United States Jaycees. (1975). All in the family: Understanding how we teach and influence children about alcohol. Participants' workbook and chairman's guide. Tulsa, OK: Author.

See No. 491.

* Warner, R. (1973). Preventing drug abuse: Where are we now? Personnel and Guidance Journal, 51 (8), 523-529.

See No. 367.

66. Wilson, W. and Helm, S. (1970). An alcoholism program tailored to community needs. Hospital and community psychiatry, 21 (12), 406-408.

Describes a treatment program that has success with alcoholics and drug addicts. The developers of this program contend that when a program reflects the needs of those being treated, clients will more frequently seek it out. The staff training of this program is a key element in the programs success.

67. Wonacott, M. and Krause, S. (1984). Combat problems of student chemical use. Module E-10 of category E-Instructional Management. Professional teacher education module series. Columbus, OH: Ohio State University, National Center for Research in Vocational Education.

Presents a learning package, one in a series, that focuses on a specific skill that vocational educators need to be successful in the area of instructional management. The purpose of this module is to prepare teachers to deal with students who are using drugs.

68. Worden, Mark. (1981). Learning how to use drugs safely. Grassroots, 9(3/81).

Presents unique approach to prevention strategies. Unique in that it focuses on the sociological aspects of substance abuse.

School Administrators' Guides

* Allen, L. and others. (1976). Health education for special children: Primary EMR. Albany, NY: New York State Education Department.

See No. 417.

69. American Association for Health, Physical Education, and Recreation. (1969). Research book for drug abuse information. Washington, DC: National Science Teachers Association.

Presents materials about teaching about drugs, facts about drugs, and supplemental reports that deal with prevention, drug use and student value correlates, motivation, etc. The section that deals with teaching about drugs presents practical and concrete suggestions for elementary and secondary school teachers, as well as administrators. Much of the focus is communication with youth.

70. Barrins, P. (1970). How to face drug abuse in your schools and your community. American school board, 158 (2), 26.

Describes the need for school boards to begin recognizing the drug abuse problem in our nation's school systems and suggests that they set up programs to respond to these issues.

71. Bay-Borelli, M., and others. (1981). Attainable alternatives: Decisions for the 80's. A district manual on substance use, abuse, and prevention. Cortland, NY: Cortland-Madison Board of Cooperative Education.

Presents a manual designed to help school personnel assess the extent of substance abuse and to develop policies and procedures for dealing with the problem through the cooperation of schools, parents, and communities. Roles and responsibilities of school personnel are outlined, including curriculum considerations and objectives. A wide variety of preventive programs are discussed in detail with names and addresses of resource groups and organizations.

* Carlisle Area School District. (1970). A program for the prevention of drug abuse: Kindergarten-Adult. Carlisle, PA: Author.

See No. 3.

* Center of Alcohol Studies. (1980). Recent topics in alcohol studies. Piscataway, NJ: Rutgers University.

See No. 589.

* Coleman, J. (1978). Deviant subcultures and the schools. In: Theoretical perspectives on school crime. Vol. I. Washington, DC: Department of Health, Education and Welfare.

See No. 501.

72. Conroy, G., and Brayer, H. (1978). Teen involvement for drug abuse prevention. Administrators' guide. (Report No. DHEW-ADM-78-624). Rockville, MD: National Institute of Drug Abuse.

Describes the Teen Involvement Program, a prevention program that is primarily implemented by youth, with guidance and direction from qualified, concerned adults. It aims at prevention through youth-to-youth communications. Junior and senior high school students are trained to discuss causes of drug abuse and ways of preventing it with students in grades 4-12. This monograph describes ways in which school administrators may develop this program in their school.

73. Davis, R. (1973). Mental Health Program for Sacramento Unified School District Elementary School Principals. Practicum report in partial fulfillment of National Ed.D. Program for educational leaders, Nova University. Sacramento, CA: Author.

Reports on the development of a professionally prepared and delivered mental health program that addresses the needs and interest of elementary principals in a Califorina school district.

74. Jackson, D. (1971). Drug Abuse: How can Boards deal with it? Evanston, IL: National School Boards Association.

Examines how school boards often view the drug problem, its prevention and the educating and helping of users. Explores baises and prejudices concerning drug use and users as well as critically reviewing educational and preventive measures.

* Mills, K., Neal, E., and Peed-Neal, I. (1983). Handbook for alcohol education: The community approach. Cambridge, MA: Ballinger.

See No.283.

* Moskowitz, J., Schaps, E., Schaeffer, G., and Malvin, J. (1984). Evaluation of a substance abuse prevention program for junior high school students. International journal of the addictions, 19 (4), 419-430.

See No. 290.

75. National Highway Traffic Safety Administration. (1984). The best prevention: Model alcohol and drug education program. NHTSA Prevention Guide. Washington, DC: Author.

Presents a guide developed for school administrators, parents, teachers, and community groups interested in developing effective alcohol and drug prevention programs for elementary and secondary schools. It describes a comprehensive approach to school-based prevention programs.

* National Institute on Alcohol Abuse and Alcoholism. (1984). Prevention plus: Involving schools, parents, and the community in alcohol and drug education. Rockville, MD: Author.

See No. 13.

76. New York State Education Dept. (1970). Guidelines for school programs in the prevention of drug abuse. Albany, NY: Author.

Provides programmatic and realistic suggestions for the development by schools of successful drug abuse prevention services.

77. Nickerson, C. (1973). The secondary school principal and student drug use. NASSP bulletin, 57(372), 55-65.

Describes what the author refers to as a "lack of sophistication" that marks our efforts to combat drug abuse. He suggests that school administrators consider the complex relationships among the individual, drugs, and society in creating effective drug education programs.

* Spivak, H. (1978). Health problems in the elementary school. National elementary principal, 57(2), 19-22.

See No. 338.

* Texas Education Agency, Austin Division of Crime Prevention and Drug Education. (1975). Administrators' handbook for crime prevention and drug education. Austin, TX: Author.

See No. 486.

78. Texas Education Agency, Austin Division of Crime Prevention and Drug Education. (1973). A framework for crime prevention and drug education in Texas: Desirable student outcomes. Austin, TX: Author.

Presents the findings of a two-year study by staff members of the Texas Education Agency for the prevention of crime and drug abuse in schools. It presents a guide to assist school personnel in organizing and implementing a sequential program of instruction in crime prevention and drug education. It is a useful guide in the planning and evaluation of prevention programs.

* U.S. Department of Health and Human Services. (1980). Beyond the three R's: Training teachers for affective education. Rockville, MD: Author.

See No. 357.

YOUTH AND PREVENTION

Program Development

79. Addiction Research Foundation. (1979). Core knowledge in the drug field. Ontario, Canada: Author.

    Contains a 12-part set of writings on the many aspects of drug abuse treatment, education, prevention, economics, etiology, history and pharmacology.

80. Aguirre, M. (1978). I.D.E.A. Alcohol Education Handbook. New York, NY: East Harlem Council for Human Services.

    Describes activities, educational endeavors, and strategies for imparting alcohol awareness and information to urban youth.

* Anderson, D., and Gadaleto, A. (1976). That happy feeling-An innovative model for a campus alcohol education program. Ratford, VA: Ratford University.

    See No. 1.

* Appleby, A. (1981, March). Alternatives for adolescents. In:Proceedings of the First Pan-Pacific Conference on Drugs and Alcohol. Canberra, Australia.

    See No. 374.

81. Archer, E., and Arundell, R. (1978). A measuring instrument for use in drug education programs: Development of the McLeod High Risk Inventory. Journal of drug education, 8(4), 313-325.

Discusses the development of an evaluation tool that is designed to test the statistical relationship between a number of psychological states and pro-drug attitudes or frequent drug use. The instrument is also designed to measure the effectiveness of drug abuse prevention.

82. Aubrey, R. (1970). Observations on the current drug scene. Journal of the National Association of College Admissions Counselors, 15 (3), 24-26.

Presents a 10-point program stating key elements which the author suggests can and should be developed to coordinate activities of the school and community towards more effective prevention efforts.

* Babst, D., Miran, M., and Kaval, M. (1976). The relationship between friends' marijuana use, family cohesion, school interest, and drug abuse prevention. Journal of drug education, 6 (1), 23-39.

See No. 418.

83. Bell, E. (1980). Content analysis of teenaged interviews for designing drug programs. Journal of drug education, 10 (2), 173-179.

Analyses of the data and youths' prescriptions concerning prevention of abuse yielded 12 program recommendations. These programs can create the awareness that leads to concerted programs to stop war and pollution. When designing educational-information programs, one must be aware of the total systems of casual factors.

84. Braucht, G. (1975). Preventing teenage problem drinking: An enticing prospect, tried but unproven. Psychiatric opinion, 12 (3), 22-25.

Examines the effectiveness of preventive efforts which have been primarily legal programs and educational programs. The authors suggest that the data indicate that all substance abuse problems are only one of a class of socially deviant behaviors, all of which are rooted in sociocultural and personal factors. It is concluded that there is a need to develop a normative sense of both adult and adolescent alcohol use and that a means of early identification of problem drinkers needs to be developed.

85. Caliguri, J. (1975). Educational policy and the drug problem: A redistributive politics issue. Journal of drug education, 5 (4), 293-300.

Describes the drug abuse problem as a cluster of problems affecting broad interests and groups. The author contends that one method of solving these problems is through a redistributive effort. The author recommends that policies and programs need to be developed as well as genuine citizen participation in the formulation of these policies.

* Center of Alcohol Studies. (1980). Recent topics in alcohol studies. Piscataway, NJ: Rutgers University.

See No. 589.

86. Cohen, A. (1973). Alternatives to drug abuse: Steps toward prevention. Rockville, MD: National Institute on Drug Abuse.

Describes a variety of alternatives to drug abuse and the problems generally associated with initial drug use: boredom, alienation, pain, frustration, and meaninglessness. The material is designed for educators, community groups, drug abuse professionals, treatment personnel, parents, and young people.

87. Conte, A., and Mason, E. (1970). Drug abuse: A challenge for education. Trenton, NJ: New Jersey Urban Schools Development Council.

Provides comprehensive information about drug use and abuse in the schools. It specifies devoted to a state-by-state description of the prevention programs in that state. It further explores available treatment resources.

88. Cross, D. (1981, July). Prevention Strategies. Paper presented at the 7th Annual Illinois Teenage Institute on Substance Abuse, Monticello, IL.

Discusses prevention strategies as tools in controlling substance abuse. Recommendations for developing and implementing prevention programs are given.

89. Davidson, F., and Manciaux, M. (1983). Alcohol and youth: What are the priorities for prevention? In: O. Jeanneret, (Ed.), Alcohol and youth. Basel, Switzerland: S. Karger.

Describes prevention objectivies and delineates requisites for prevention programs.

90. Delgado, M. and Humm-Delgado, D. (1983). Hispanic adolescents and substance abuse: Issues for the 1980s. In: R. Isralowitz, and M. Singer (Eds.), Adolescent Substance Abuse: A guide to prevention and treatment. New York, NY: Haworth Press.

Attempts to describe the status of drug and alcohol abuse among the Hispanic youth and to identify issues which researchers, clinicians, administrators, etc., will have to address in the 80's. Suggests that attention be given to culture-specific prevention programs.

91. Dembo, R., and Burgos, W. (1976). A framework for developing drug abuse prevention strategies for young people in ghetto areas. Journal of drug education, 6(4), 313-323.

Describes a model of prevention activities for ghetto youth. Developed using research and literature on socialization, social psychology, and drug abuse. This is an ethnographically informed, social context model.

92. Dembo, R., and Miran, M. (1975). Evaluation of drug prevention programs by youths in a middle class community. International journal of the addictions, 11(5).

Examines young peoples' reactions to various prevention programs and reports program topics that the authors would like to see included in future prevention efforts.

93. Douglas, R. (1982). Youth, alcohol, and traffic accidents. In: Alcohol and Health Mono. No. 4: Special Population Issues. Washington, DC: United States Government Printing Office.

Discusses the role that alcohol plays in traffic accidents. Describes alcohol related accidents as the most frequent cause of death and disability of American youth. Makes recommendations for prevention efforts in this area.

94. Drug Abuse Council, Inc. (1972). Survey of state drug abuse activities 1972. (Report No.: MS-2). Washington, DC: Author

Presents a survey that was one of a series to explain the efforts of the public sector to control and prevent drug abuse. Contains a census of existing programs and expenditures, as well as a review of unmet problems and needs. The report includes an analysis of the possible problems developing in these efforts by the various states to respond to drug abuse.

95. Ebel, H. (1975). Effect of a marijuana drug-education program: Comparison of faculty-elicited and student-elicited data. Journal of drug education, 5(1), 77-85.

Presents a study that examines the effects of a drug education course on the relationship between drug attitudes and usage, and the validity of attitude and usage relations. The study was conducted through a comparison evaluation elicited by peers and teachers.

96. Educational Commission of the States. (1974). Task force on responsible decisions about alcohol, Interim Report Number 1. Summary document and reports on working conferences. Denver, CO: Author.

Describes a program designed to totally involve the educational system in the efforts to combat drug abuse. The task force determined that alcoholism is a reaction to daily living situations, suggested reasons why prevention efforts have fallen short, explored the relationship of decision-making to alcohol abuse, and the effect of the human services programs on alcohol use and abuse. No clear assessment of how genetic, physiological, psychological, and societal factors influence the problem, nor any reasons for present prevention services having had limited effectiveness on the problem are presented.

* Fontan, M. (1983, August). Principles of prevention. In: Proceedings of the Fourth World Congress for the Prevention of Alcoholism and Drug Dependency. Nairobi, Kenya: Author.

See No. 206.

97. Frank, P. (1978). Drug abuse is alive and well. Education forum, 42(4), 459-467.

The author argues that drug abuse prevention has failed. He concludes that children need early decision making opportunities to form values, and describes how drug use and abuse are promoted by intensive industry advertising

98. General Research Corp. (1973). Evaluation of selected components of the Office of Education "Help Communities Help Themselves" drug abuse prevention program. Washington, DC: United States Department of Health, Education and Welfare.

Presents a program, Help Communities Help Themselves, a community based drug abuse prevention program. Describes the evaluation process, needs assessment and development of the program. In addition, it suggests developmental tasks for youth that are viewed by the author as healthy and appropriate. The authors suggest that the failure of many prevention efforts is the result of having inappropriate expectations for youth.

99. Glynn, T., and others (Eds.). Preventing adolescent drug abuse: Intervention strategies. NIDA Research Monograph 47. A RAUS Review Report. Rockville, MD: National Institute on Drug Abuse.

Presents a collection of papers which begins with a presentation on the role of mass media campaigns in drug abuse prevention, emphasizing the need for skill development and family involvement. Other papers focus on issues of family, peers, school, and the individual. A three-dimensional model is presented for prevention.

* Griffin, T., and Svendsen, R. (1980). Student Assistance Program: How it works. Center City, MN: Hazeldon Foundation.

See No. 32.

100. Goldstein, J. (1974). Students' evaluations of their psychoactive drug use. New York: Carnegie Mellon Unversity.

Presents findings of a longitudinal study of self-reported surveys concerning psychoactive drug use over the four year period of 1968 to 1972.

101. Heidenreich, C. (1976). Alcohol and drug abuse and use among Indian-Americans: A review of issues and sources. Journal of drug issues, 6(3), 256-272.

Presents alcohol and drug abuse as being among the top problems in the United States in general and also a high priority health and social problem among Indians. Reviews litera-

literature and presents an overview of some of the major perspectives that should be included in any program being developed to serve this population. Suggestions are made for programs, services and prevention strategies.

102. Hewitt, L. (1982). Current status of alcohol education programs for youth. In: Alcohol and health mono. no. 4: Special populations. Washington, DC: U.S. Government Printing Office.

Describes alcohol prevention programs as they appear in the literature since the 70's. The author contends that these methods are still viable as an approach to prevention.

* Hochhauser, M. (1981). Ethical issues in academic substance abuse consultation. Paper presented at the 89th Annual Convention of the American Psychological Association, Los Angeles, CA.

See No. 36.

103. Huba, G., Wingard, J., and Bentler, P. (1980). Applications of a theory of drug use to prevention programs. Journal of drug education, 10(1), 25-37.

Outlines an interactive theory of drug use and provides the framework for integrating current knowledge and initiating new research on prevention issues. The model is presented as an evolutionary one which will grow as new data and clinical experiences are collected.

104. Jacobs, P. (1977, September). A rural community's response to drug abuse. Paper presented at the Rural Sociological Society Annual Meeting, Madison, WI.

Describes a program developed to combat the continued growth of drug and alcohol abuse in a rural community. The program is built upon an educational/preventive drug treatment program including, in addition to networks to other providers, individual, group, and family counseling; drug education to schools and community; criminal justice referral/ intake; drug diversion and prevention; crisis intervention; speakers' bureau; recreation services; and a hot line for clients in need.

* Jaynes, J., and Rugg, C. (1983). Role of chemical abuse during adolescence. Focus on alcohol and drug issues, 6(3), 16-17.

See No. 387.

* Johnson, N. (1982). Michigan develops curriculum to reduce DWI among youth. Alcohol, health and research world. 7(1), 35-37.

See No. 241.

105. Kaiser, L. (Ed.). (1983). Chemical people book. Pittsburgh, PA: QED Enterprises.

Describes the conceptualization, design, and implementation of "The Chemical People," a media bound, community outreach, prevention, and education effort. Discusses the role of community resources, parents, schools, social support systems, etc., in the overall effort. Suggestions for prevention strategies are given that may be adopted by various communities.

106. Kaplonek, W. (1977, June). Clarification of systematic materials on youth protection from stimulant abuse. Paper presented at the 23rd International Institute on Prevention and Treatment of Alcoholism. Dresden, Germany.

Describes the efforts of the East German Youth Organization to prevent drug abuse.

107. Killinger, G., and others. (1974). Selected papers by Institute Faculty. Criminal justice monograph, VII. No I. Huntsville, TX: Sam Houston University.

Presents 12 papers on the subjects of delinquency prevention, drug abuse prevention, prevention alternatives, treatment alternatives, and counseling issues. All authors write from a sociological background, some from experience in the criminal justice system.

108. Kleinot, M., and Rogers, R. (1982). Identifying effective components of alcohol misuse prevention programs. Journal of studies on alcohol, 43(7), 802-811.

Tested three main components of many informal programs for the prevention of alcohol misuse and alcoholism. Implications for program design are noted.

109. Larsen, B., Krynak, D., and Pettyjohn, T. (1981). Alcohol and other drug use among rural adolescents: Some implications for rural drug programming. In: A.J. Schecter (Ed.), Drug dependency and alcoholism, Vol. 2: Social behavior issues. New York, NY: Plenum Press.

Presents data from a survey conducted to obtain baseline data on the extent and patterns of alcohol and drug use among teenagers in rural Ohio. The authors note that the significance of the study lies in the capability for joint agency/school use of the data for short and long term program planning efforts, education/prevention, and treatment/counseling.

110. Lassey, M., and Carlson, J. (1981). Teenage drinking in Idaho's rural communities. Moscow, ID: University of Idaho College of Agriculture.

Examines teenage drinking in a rural region of Idaho. Explores factors that lead teenagers to drink including peer pressure and family influences. Describes possible alternatives to teenage drinking, including alcohol education programs that include parents, school programs, peer counseling, and mass media development.

* Link, W., and others. (1979). Drugs in prespective: Trainers manual and resource guide. Gaithersburg, MD: National Drug Abuse Center for Training and Resource Development.

See No. 41.

111. Lynch, M. (1967). "US": Primary prevention, para-counseling, research project. Rockville, MD: National Institute on Drug Abuse.

Presents a program that was developed with funding from the National Institute on Drug Abuse to design a model prevention program that could be replicated nationwide. Describes the training of volunteer staff, program development, and final evaluation of program effects on participants.

112. Mathews, W. (1974). A critique of traditional drug education programs. Paper presented at the Annual Meeting of the American Educational Research Association. Chicago, IL.

Presents a critical look at drug education prevention efforts to date of publication. Describes the strategies of drug education efforts as two broad categories: the supporting mode and the converting mode. The author contends that neither of these efforts have had much success and presents considerations and suggestions for drug educators.

113. Messolonghites, L. (Ed.). (1974). Alternative pursuits for America's 3rd century: A resource book on new perceptions, processes, and programs with implications for the prevention of drug abuse. Rockville, MD: National Institute on Drug Abuse.

Describes some of the more frequent reasons for drug abuse and the use of an alternatives approach as a means of prevention. Includes selections from literature on drug abuse prevention and strategies for prevention that support the validity for the alternatives approach. Selections include, among others, the following topics: new trends, strategies, institution processes, values, lifestyles, attitudes, points of view, and programs.

114. Mills, K., and McCarthy, D. (1983). A data-based alcohol abuse prevention program in a university setting. Journal of alcohol and drug education, 28(2), 15-27.

Presents a formal design for a prevention program that can be developed as part of any college or university. Details for program evaluation are included.

115. Milner, G. (1977). The treatment of alcoholic and drug dependent persons in Victoria. Journal of drug issues, 7(4), 385-389.

Summarizes the development of a multidisciplinary, community oriented treatment, research, and rehabilitation program for alcoholics and drug abusers. May be valuable as a secondary prevention model for youthful substance abusers.

* Monroe-Scott, B., and Miranda, V. (1981). Guidebook for planning alcohol prevention programs with black youth. Rockville, MD: Clearinghouse for Alcohol Information.

See No. 384.

116. Morriss, R. (1983) . Peer education teaches Minnesota teenagers the control factor in drinking and driving. Traffic Safety, 83 (5), 6-8.

Describes a peer education program that was developed to lessen the number of accidents involving youth that had been drinking. The author concludes that the program did not meet its stated objectives.

117. Moser, J. (1980). Prevention of alcohol related problems. Toronto, Canada: Addiction Research Foundation Marketing Services.

Reviews international preventive measures,

policies, and programs. Contributors are from more than 80 countries from six member regions of the World Health Organization. Provides a cultural and legal perspective of the problem and a source for research for professionals in the field.

118. Nail, R., and Gunderson, E. (1975). The youthful drug abuser and drug abuse education: Closing the credibility gap. Journal of drug education, 5(1), 65-75.

Notes that increasing evidence supports the contention that most drug prevention efforts are ineffective. The authors refer this criticism to both individual school efforts as well as federal projects. A brief statement of the state of the art of prevention programs is included. Five major classes of drug users are noted as well as seven primary objectives for future program development efforts to include. Concludes that evidence calls for an unemotional and honest approach to drug abuse, thus allowing rational youth to deal with the issues at an individual level.

119. National Drug Center for Training and Resources Development. (1981). Community based prevention specialist. Participant Manual. Bethesda, MD: University Research Corporation.

Describes skills required to assist substance abuse prevention specialists in the development of knowledge and skills in implementing community based programs through an entry level course. Presents nine training modules and the required materials, exercises, and activities related to these. The course materials focus towards prevention strategies, knowledge of the community, the development of community support, implementation techniques, and prevention of staff burnout.

and the community in alcohol and drug education. Rockville, MD: Author.

See No. 13.

120. National Institute on Drug Abuse. (1980). The Learning Laboratory. Services Research Monograph Series. Rockville, MD: Author.

Presents curriculum and program development materials for a community based education program that has incorporated prevention strategies into the overall approach to remediation and education.

121. New York State Division of Alcoholism and Alcohol Abuse (DAAA). (1986). Focus on prevention-5 year comprehensive plan for alcohol services in New York State, 1984-1989. Albany, NY: Author

Presents prevalence data, prevention strategies, prevention initiatives, for school, community, and local government action. Types of program services are outlined. Specific attention is placed on programs and services needed to address current prevalence data.

122. Noll, A. (1974). "Drug abuse and its prevention" as seen by the international legal profession: Report on the XIth International Congress on Penal Law. Bulletin on narcotics, 27(1), 37-47

Discusses the subjects reviewed at the congress including the nature and trends of substance abuse, prospective legislation, law enforcement issues, treatment and rehabilitation of abusers, international control and prevention efforts

123. Norem-Hebeisen, A., Ardyth A., and Lucas, M. (1977). A developmental model for primary prevention of chemical abuse. Journal of drug education, 7(2), 141-147.

Proposes a developmental model that suggests

five concurrent perspectives for developing curriculum with a goal of prevention of chemical abuse. The five perspectives provide the basis for a hierarchy of instructional objectives.

124. North Carolina State Department of Public Instruction. (1974). Resource books for values education. Raleigh, NC: Author.

Cites resource books on the philosophy, purpose, and methods of values education. Also cited are workshop guides for the learning of value clarification techniques by parents, and a series of curriculum guides designed for a drug abuse prevention program.

* Overend, R. (1982). You can say no to alcohol: Government media campaign for teens and women. Traffic safety, 8(4), 18-20.

See No. 299.

125. Pickover, B., Barbrack, C., and Glat, M. (1982). Preventive and educative programs within the high school. School psychology review, 11(4), 399-408.

Presents a literature review indicating that school psychologists have been minimally involved in sex, drug, and vocational education, as well as the teaching of psychology courses in high school. The question of the effectiveness of drug education programs is discussed in terms of the roles the school psychologist may maintain through the program planning process.

126. Pringle, H., Gregory, J., Ginkel, K. and Cheek, C. (1981). Alpha centers: A viable prevention model for substance abuse agencies and public schools. In: A.J. Schecter (Ed.), Drug dependency and alcoholism, Vol. 2: Social behavior issues. New York, NY: Plenum Press.

Describes the Alpha Center model for substance abuse prevention. This is a school-based prevention effort that focuses on maladaptive behaviors in the school setting and the home. The goals of this program are to develop better social and academic skills. In addition, teachers receive in-service education in classroom management techniques.

* Ramsey, G., and Barnes, L. (1976, May). Drugs, society and personal choice: A summer school for teachers. Paper presented at the Annual Convention of the Canadian Guidance and Counseling Association, Halifax, Nova Scotia.

See No. 54.

127. Regional Health Planning Council of the North Central Texas Council of Governments. (1975). Proposed 1975 North Central Texas regional plan for the prevention and treatment of alcohol abuse and alcoholism: A summary. Arlington, TX: Author.

Presents an approach for prevention and treatment services for a 16-county area of Central Texas. Includes goals, objectives, strategies, implementation and evaluation. Plan objectives include education and prevention, development of a continuous planning mechanism, and the improvement of treatment services, etc.

* Reinhart, R. (1974). The family drug awareness group: A citizen initiated example of effective community concern. Journal of drug education, 4(2), 151-155.

See No. 583.

128. Robin, F. (1976). Education in action, school year 1975-1976. Brooklyn, NY: New York City Board of Education, Office of Evaluation.

Presents an evaluation of a New York City school-based program on drug abuse prevention, the New York City Umbrella Programs. The project included a community health education effort that focused on parents as well as students. An analysis of the results indicate that staff and parents achieved mastery of the materials covered but the author makes no reference to behavioral change.

129. Robins, L. (1974, May). The Vietnam drug user returns. Final report. Special action office monograph, Series A, No. 2. Rockville, MD: United States Government Printing Office.

Presents the findings of a survey of 965 servicemen returning from Vietnam. The report includes the returnees' suggestions as to how the army should cope with widespread drug use, prevention efforts, and the types of services needed by veterans.

130. Ryan, W., and Hettena, C. (1976). Project youth: An approach to drug abuse. Elementary school guidance and counseling, 10(4), 270-278.

Describes a drug prevention program for preadolescent children. The program tends to achieve its aims through the use of small group work and positive peer influence, development of positive self-concept, and problem solving skills. Evaluation shows that it is influential in changing student characteristics.

131. Samuels, D., and Samuels, M. (1975). The complete handbook of peer counseling. An authorative guide for the organization, training, implementation and evaluation of a peer counseling program. Miami, FL: Fiesta Publishing.

Describes the advantages of peer counseling within a drug education and prevention program. Stresses its advantage over traditional prevention models. Describes in detail the procedures for developing, implementing, and evaluation a peer counseling/prevention model program.

132. Schinke, S., and others. (1985). Strategies for preventing substance abuse with American Indian youth. <u>White cloud journal of American Indian mental health</u>, 3(4), 12-18.

Suggests strategies for assessment, design, implementation, and evaluation of substance abuse prevention programs with American Indian youth. Illustrates use of each strategy with examples from drug abuse prevention activities in Northwest Indian communities.

* Seabright, C. (1973). A look at some current programs. <u>Journal of drug education</u>, 3 (2), 127-140.

See No. 328.

133. Selin, J., and Svanum, S. (1981). Alcoholism and substance abuse training: A survey of graduate programs in clinical psychology. <u>Professional psychology</u>, <u>12</u>(6), 717-721.

Surveyed the A.P.A.'s approved clinical psychology programs in an attempt to quantify the extent of research activity, clinical course work, and training offered or required in the areas of alcoholism and drug abuse. Findings indicate that there is a low priority on training in these areas in the graduate schools.

134. Social Advocates for Youth. (1978). <u>Early age prevention of alcohol abuse project: Final report</u>. San Francisco, CA: Author.

Describes and provides an overview of the essential elements of a project on early age prevention of alcohol abuse. Also described is the nature and focus of other prevention efforts that are conducted by the Social Advocates for Youth. A guide to others who wish to develop similar projects is provided.

* Soroka, J. (1973). Coping with Newark's drug abuse dilemma. <u>Journal of school health</u>, <u>43</u>(2), 126-128.

See No. 337.

135. Stephen, M., and Prentice, R. (1979). Developing an occupational drug abuse program: Considerations and approaches. Services research monograph series. Ann Arbor, MI: University of Michigan Institute for Social Research.

Describes a program for the development of corporate drug abuse treatment and prevention programs. Has some relevant materials for adolescent program development in that it describes various policies and program descriptions.

136. Stenmark, D., Walfish, S., and Brennan, A. (1981). A three-course sequence in substance abuse prevention at the baccalaureate level. Teaching of psychology, 8(2), 82-85.

Describes undergraduate courses that are geared both for students who wish to specialize in this field as well as those that just have a general interest. The authors note that for students entering this field, social skills training is necessary.

* Stolz, P., and Van Der Heide, G. (1983, May). School/Community intervention workshop: A workshop on the CADAP (Community Alcohol and Drug Abuse Prevention). Paper presented at the National Drug Institute, Brisbane, Australia. Brisbane, Australia: National Drug Institute.

See No. 23.

137. Storm, T., and Cutler, R. (1975). The role of research in alcohol and drug education. Journal of alcohol and drug education, 20(2), 5-11.

Outlines several general roles for research in educational campaigns for the prevention of drug abuse. Although drug and alcohol abuse programs emphasize education as a major approach to prevention and control, there is a paucity of research on the effectiveness of educational campaigns. The authors note that a major role for research in the planning and conducting of these campaigns is objective evaluation for the purpose of discovering what elements in a program are effective and how to increase this effectiveness.

138. Sugarman, B., and Lachapelle, C. (1975). Drug abuse and the community: A model for the effective coordination of prevention, control, and treatment resources. Drug forum, 4(4), 295-309.

Presents a model of the basic components necessary in a comprehensive community program to combat drug abuse. These components are defined as prevention, treatment, control or law enforcement, and coordination or policy making.

139. Swisher, J., and others. (1976). Hispanic mental health, drugs and alcohol policy issues: Views from the field. Coral Gables, FL: University of Miami.

Presents three papers from a conference held for the purpose of examining the status of health and human services among Hispanic Americans. The problem of drug abuse is described as a symptom of dysfunctional family structures, a problem created by pressures to adapt within the American social context. Recommendations are made for drug abuse prevention from an integrated strategy including training, legislation, treatment and research.

* Texas Education Agency, Austin Division of Crime Prevention and Drug Education. (1973). A framework for crime prevention and drug education in Texas: Desirable student outcomes. Austin, TX: Author.

See No. 78.

141. U.S. Department of Education. (1986). What works--Schools without drugs. Washington, DC: Author.

Presents readings on the prevalence of

substance abuse in the schools, makes suggestions for parental responses, school system responses, and student responses. It further suggests some curriculum and gives a resource section for further information on services and other relevant materials.

* U.S. Department of Health and Human Services. (1981). The Door: A model youth center. Rockville, MD: Author.

See No. 358.

* Ventura, M., and Dundon, M. (1974). A challenging experience in canoeing and camping as a tool in approaching the drug problem. Journal of drug education, 4(1), 123-127.

See No. 361.

* Vejnoska, J. (1982). Parent action groups: A prevention resource. Alcohol Health and Research World, 6(4), 13-17.

See No. 362.

* Warner, R. (1973). Preventing drug abuse: Where are we now? Personnel and Guidance Journal, 5.1(8), 523-529.

See No. 367.

* West, P., and others. (1976). Report on a needs assessment and evaluation of a drug education program. Van Nuys, CA: Los Angeles Valley College.

See No. 369.

142. Wheeler, W. (1976). Blackness is my mental health: A mind set for black drug abuse prevention and treatment programs. Journal of non-white concerns in personnel and guidance, 4(2), 64-70.

Discusses the factors responsible for the failure of programs aimed at eliminating drug abuse, especially in the black community. He feels that the existing social and political system and those blacks who cooperate with it are responsible for this failure.

143. Wiener, R. (1971). A report on a drug education program. Journal of drug education, 1(4), 305-315.

Describes a drug education program developed in the Netherlands. This program used three different approaches: mild horror, factual, and individual adjustment.

* Wilson, W., and Helm, S. (1970). An alcoholism program tailored to community needs. Hospital and community psychiatry, 21(12), 406-408.

See No. 66.

* Wong, M. (1975, April). Different strokes: Models of drug abuse prevention. Paper presented at the Annual Meeting of the American Educational Research Association, Washington, DC.

See No. 372.

Program Evaluations/Reviews

144. Abt Associates, Inc. (1982). An evaluation of the impact of employment specialists in drug abuse treatment. Treatment research report. Cambridge, MA: Author.

Findings indicate that programs that employed full-time employment specialists as part of the treatment staff were more successful both in retaining clients in treatment as well as achieving a higher rate of success upon completion of the program.

145. ADAMA. (1983). Preventing adolescent drug abuse: Intervention strategies. NIDA research monograph no. 47: RAUS review report. Rockville, MD: Author.

Presents papers and discussions based on the Research Analysis and Utilization System (RAUS) on strategies for the prevention of adolescent drug abuse. Contains a summary of discussions and recommendations.

146. Adams, R., Benjamin, M., Berberian, R., and Kline, G. (1977). Alcoholism prevention and treatment services in counties: Report on a national survey. Rockville, MD: National Institute on Alcohol Abuse and Alcoholism.

Describes a national survey that attempted to assess the efforts of counties in providing alcoholism prevention and treatment services. Discusses program planning, funding, program coordination, and other related subjects. Other topics include criminal justice involvement, occupational alcohol programming, and some of the major obstacles to the provision of services.

147. Alcoholic Liquor Advisory Council. (1980). Alcohol and you. Wellington, New Zealand: Author.

Presents facts and information for youth about drinking and alcohol. Exercises are provided to enhance the reader's knowledge of this information.

148. Alcoholism and the Hispanic: A mutual concern. El alcoholismo y los hispanos una preocupacion nacional. (1981, September). Proceedings of the National Hispanic Conference on Alcoholism, San Antonio, TX.

Conference papers emphasizing recommendations for remediation of alcohol-related problems, including prevention programs.

149. American Justice Institute. (1971). Juvenile drug abuse prevention project. Santa Clara County Juvenile Probation Department. First year evaluation report. Sacramento, CA: Author.

Presents the evaluation of a court diversion project developed to refer juveniles with drug abuse backgrounds to appropriate treatment providers. Appendices contain type of data collected, data analysis procedure, and supporting data not contained in the text.

150. Anastas, R. (1982, August). Prepared statement for the U.S. Senate Committee on Alcoholism and Drug Abuse. U.S. Senate Hearing on Alcohol, Drugs and Driving. Washington, DC: United State Government Printing Office.

Presents statistical information on the prevalence of alcohol related traffic accidents. The program, Students Against Driving Drunk (SADD), is described.

151. Baiterman, M. (1982). Youth and alcohol: Is there really an epidemic? Journal of alcohol and drug education, 28(1), 43-52.

Addresses the question of whether or not there is truly an epidemic of adolescent alcoholism. Focuses on a variety of youth-oriented topics. Describes various prevention and intervention strategies as well as some of the difficulties of providing services to adolescent clients.

152. Barbara, J. (1982). Law enforcement and substance abuse prevention: Training and strategy selection. Journal of drug education, 12(1), 29-42.

Describes a training program and a specific information strategy for police promoting substance abuse prevention. Discusses training components for a successful drug abuse presentation and selection of an appropriate prevention strategy. Presents a model of types of drug information. Discusses problems with negative attitudes and use of drug surveys.

153. Barkin, A. (1983, February). Teenage alcohol abuse prevention in New England. Paper presented at the Meeting of Teenage Alcohol Abuse Prevention Programs. Sturbridge, MA.

Presents a prevention program that has been referred to as successful in the prevention of adolescent alcohol abuse.

154. Barnes, G. (1984). Evaluation of alcohol education: A reassessment using socialization theory. Journal of drug education, 14(2), 133-150.

Argues that the design and evaluation of alcohol education and prevention programs should be guided by social theory in order to establish the most appropriate goals, methods, and interpretations of program outcomes. The author suggests that, to date, prevention programs have offered little to no help in the changing of behaviors, attitudes or substance abuse patterns of our youth.

155. Barnes, R., and others. (1984). An evaluation of a youth awareness program (YAP),

school year 1983-84. Washington, DC: District of Columbia Public Schools.

Evaluates the Youth Awareness Program, a joint effort of District of Columbia Public Schools and the Metropolitan Police Department, which focuses on helping high school students make appropriate decisions about sex, drugs, crime, and careers, as well as motivating students toward positive behaviors.

156. Bayh, B. (1975). Our nation's schools--A report card: "A" in school violence and vandalism. Preliminary report of the subcommittee to investigate juvenile delinquency. Washington, DC: Congress of the U.S., Senate Committee on the Judiciary.

Presents the findings of the above-mentioned subcommittee's work on drug abuse prevention, runaway youth, delinquency, school dropouts. The Committee gathered testimony from 419 witnesses who addressed the issues from the years 1970 to 1975.

157. Beaupre, R. (1981). Commentary to Interface: The Health and Justice Systems. In: Addictions: What is their treatment? Conference proceedings. Ottawa, Canada: Commoners Publications.

Discusses the economic effects of substance abuse and stresses the need for prevention measures to combat these problems.

158. Bell, E. (1980). Content analysis of teenaged interviews for designing drug programs. Journal of drug education, 10(2), 173-179.

Presents recommendations that were gathered from youth on the need for and the design of prevention programs. Their suggestions for prevention programs are included.

159. Bennett, G. (1983). Youthful substance abuse. In: G. Bennett et al. (Eds.), Substance abuse: Perspectives. New York, NY: Wiley & Sons.

Presents issues related to substance abuse prevention for youth. Attempts to differentiate between use and abuse, provides a history of substance abuse, presents the scope of present and future abuse, indicates some of the factors that influence abuse, and defines some of the major approaches to prevention.

160. Berberian, R., Gross, C., Lovejoy, J., and Paperalle, S. (1976). The effectiveness of drug education programs: A critical review. Health education monographs, 4(4), 377-398.

Critiques previous findings and methods of program evaluations conducted on 27 prevention programs. The authors suggest that school based prevention programs design evaluation studies as experiments with controlled manipulation of relevant variations.

161. Bisard, M. (1974). Final report on the Youth Service Agency, the City of Rockhill, South Carolina. Rock Hill, SC: Rock Hill Planning and Management Department.

The program contains six project components for a more comprehensive approach to the problems of youth. The author concludes that most of the objectives of this program have been met and are demonstrated through lessened criminal contact for respective youth in treatment.

162. Blangiardo, J., and Gold, J. (1982). Alternative drug and alcohol prevention program. Self evaluation, 1981-82. Brooklyn, NY: Community School District 22.

Presents the evaluation results of a school-based drug and alcohol prevention program that services students, their families, and the community. This is done primarily through prevention groups; intervention services, focusing on the needs of at-risk youth; and the Alternative Class which office services to students who do not function well in the traditional class setting. The appendix contains evaluation materials, findings and recommendations for the future.

163. Blizard, R., and Teague, R. (1981). Alternatives to drug use: An alternative approach to drug education. International journal of the addictions, 16(2), 371-375.

Describes and evaluates the Alcohol and Drug Education Course, a secondary prevention program for drug-abusing adolescents. It is designed to provide drug use information as well as to present alternatives to drug and alcohol use for achieving altered states of consciousness. The program is reported to be successful in increasing the students' awareness of alternatives to drug use, and the hazards of drug abuse, and in decreasing their reported reliance on drugs for achievement of altered states of consciousness.

164. Blokker, W., Glaser-Kirschenbaum, W. and Kirschenbaum, H. (1976). Values clarification and drug abuse. Health education, 7(March/April), 6-8.

Describes an evaluation project of fourth, fifth, and sixth grade students and their response to a values clarification approach to prevention.

165. Boguslawski, A. (1981). Abstinence and pathfinders union. Problemy alkoholizmu, 28(9), 12-14.

Presents a discussion among the leaders of the Pathfinders Union, a Polish scouting group, regarding the incidence of alcohol abuse that was discovered among these youth. Recommendations for prevention efforts among similar youth are given.

166. Bosworth, K., Gustafson, D., Hawkins, R., Chewing, B., and Day, T. (1983). Adolescents, health education, and computers: The body awareness resource network (BARN). Health education, 14(6), 58-60.

Describes a computer program that is designed to act as a confidential, nonjudgmental source of health education information. Specific attention is given to drug and alcohol education. The system is designed to give support and encouragement, to maintain a positive lifestyle, as well as to provide options for choosing healthier lifestyles.

167. Botvin, G. (1983). Prevention of adolescent substance abuse through the development of personal and social competence. In: Preventing adolescent drug abuse: Intervention strategies. Rockville, MD: National Institute on Drug Abuse.

Presents the need for a prevention strategy that has a more comprehensive approach than previous models. The author calls for a model that will encompass the enhancement of personal competence through the development of basic life skills, and the acquisition of problem-specific skills, and knowledge designed to increase adolescents' abilities to resist the various forms of social pressure to smoke, drink, or use drugs.

168. Botvin, G., et al. A cognitive behavioral approach to substance abuse prevention. Addictive behaviors, 9(2), 137-147.

Presents a program that attempted to reduce intrapersonal pressure to smoke, drink excessively, or use marijuana by fostering the development of general life skills as well as teaching students tactics for resisting direct pressure to use these substances. Results indicate that the program had a significant impact on cigarette smoking, excessive drinking, and marijuana use when implemented by peer leaders.

169. Bouclans, V., and Davril, N. (1981, April). "Health Clubs" in French high schools. Paper presented at the European Youth Center Study Session, Strasbourg, France.

Describes the alcohol education program that has been offered in French High Schools since 1975.

170. Bradford, D. (1984). Alcohol and the young child. Alcohol and alcoholism, 19(2), 173-175.

Describes the incidents of alcohol poisoning of young children. The author notes that this may be imitation of parents' behaviors for children aged 3-4. Statistics and other relevant data on this subject are included.

171. Braucht, G., Follinstad, D., Brakarsh, D., and Berry, K. (1973). Drug education: A review of goals, approaches and effectiveness, and a paradigm for evaluation. Quarterly journal of studies on alcohol, 34(4), 1279-1292.

Reviews the literature on various treatment programs for youthful drinkers, drug users and prevention efforts through legal and educational means. Findings include that these efforts have not effected a decline in the incidence of alcohol or drug abusing behaviors. Suggestions for future research are made.

172. Brock, C. (1983). Serious and effective prevention strategy for the young. Digest of alcoholism theory and application, 2(3), 21-24.

Presents data from a survey designed to provide a broad base of information about knowledge, attitudes, and use patterns involving alcohol and drugs. The authors conclude that this information will assist in the development of future prevention efforts.

173. Brown, W. (1977). A skeptical look at drug education. Paper presented at the Annual Conference on Alcohol and Drug Dependence, Winnipeg, Manitoba, Canada.

Notes that attempts to provide drug abuse education have developed into a variety of programs and approaches to address this issue. The author concludes that attempts to date can be summed up as compliant behavior and are antithetical to education itself.

174. Bry, B. (1982). Reducing the incidence of adolescent problems through one and five-year follow-up. American Journal of community psychology, 10(3), 265-276.

Presents the results of a study that investigated the long term effects of a school based prevention program that had shown impressive short term success. The findings indicate that the intervention program reduced delinquency problems but the evidence was less clear for substance abuse. Future research efforts are discussed.

175. Capone, T., and others. (1973). Peer group leadership in drug abuse prevention 1970-1971 academic year. Journal of drug education, 3(3), 201-245.

Presents the evaluation of the Peer Group approach to drug abuse prevention in the New York City school system. This was a formative evaluation for an ongoing program evaluation and development, in view of this being the first year of operation for this project.

176. Carpenter, R., Lyons, C., and Miller, W. (1985). Peer-managed self-control program for prevention of alcohol abuse in American Indian high school students: A pilot evaluation study. International journal of the addictions, 20(2), 299-310.

Describes a model treatment and prevention program developed for high school students that are American Indians. It is based on the concepts of peer pressure and the idea that most abuse begins as a result of negative peer pressure and that youth respond best and quickest to other youth.

177. Center for Disease Control. (1976). The Bureau of Health Education's Elementary School Health Curriculum Project, Berkeley Model, and the American Lung Association--Bureau of Health Education's Primary Grades Health Curriculum Project, Seattle Model. Atlanta, GA: Author.

Describes two health education curriculum based projects. A unit approach to curriculum was used. The author presents selected materials, curriculum, books and films to be used. One project had a third to seventh grade focus while the other focused towards K-3.

178. Chafetz, M. (Ed.). (1973). Proceedings of the Annual Alcoholism Conference of the National Institute on Alcohol Abuse and Alcoholism (2nd), Washington, D.C., June, 1972. Psychological and social factors in drinking and treatment and treatment evaluation. Washington, DC: National Institute on Alcoholism and Alcohol Abuse.

Includes papers and research both in progress and completed. Subjects include investigations in the behavioral sciences and in particular the development of workable and effective systems of alcoholism prevention. Part I focuses on psychological and social factors, with specific attention being paid to adolescent alcoholism. Part II considers treatment and treatment evaluations.

179. Channing, L., Bete Co., Inc. (1980). What every teenager should know about alcohol. South Deerfield, MA: Author.

Presents facts for youth in regard to their decision to use alcohol or not to use alcohol.

180. Christiansen, B., Goldman, M., and Inn, A. (1982). Development of alcohol related expectancies in adolescents: Separating pharmacological from social learning influences. Journal of consulting and clinical psychology, 50(3), 336-344.

Describes the development of a questionnaire designed to distinguish pharmacological/ experiential influences from social learning influences on formation of adolescents' alcohol-related expectations. Results indicate that intervention to decrease the risk of adult problem drinking must begin with children.

181. Clark, J., et al. (1974). Operation Future: Third Annual Report. San Diego, CA: Pennant.

Describes a study that measured the effects of values clarification experiences on character traits and on students' use of drugs.

* Cohen, S. (1976). Drug use, misuse, and abuse incidents among elementary school children. Journal of drug education, 6(3), 247-251.

See No. 4.

182. Congress of the United States. (1980). Drug use and abuse in the Memphis-Shelby County School System; Hearings before the Select Committee on Narcotics Abuse and Control, House of Representatives, Ninety-Sixth Congress, Second Session. Washington, DC: United States Government Printing Office.

Contains transcripts of the hearings before the Select Committee. Presentations include those of members of the press, school system, student populations, police departments, and several mental health clinics. Statements focus on issues of prevention, treatment, the role of juvenile court systems in prevention, and student attitudes towards drug abuse among their peers.

183. Cook, R., and Morton, A. (1975). An assessment of drug education-prevention programs in the U.S. Army. Army Research Institute Technical Paper 261. Arlington, VA: Army Research Institute.

Describes the efforts by the U.S. Army in attempting to prevent drug abuse in the ranks of the Armed Forces. The data presented assess the effectiveness of these efforts. The data presented do not suggest that these programs have been successful.

184. Cook, R., Lawrence, H., Morese, C., and Roehl, J. (1984). An evaluation of the

alternatives approach to drug abuse prevention. International journal of the addictions, 19(7), 767-787.

Evaluation of a school-based drug abuse prevention program that has as its philosophy the belief that drug abuse is related to the rewards and pleasures that drug abuse provides. The authors contend that individuals must be provided with alternatives to these through the gaining of desired rewards through healthy nonchemical activities.

185. Cooper, A., and Sobell, M. (1977). Does alcohol education prevent alcohol problems?: Need for evaluation. Journal of alcohol and drug education, 25(1), 54-63.

Examines evidence for the alleged failure of alcohol education to prevent alcohol problems among children and adolescents. The authors conclude that there is a need for investigations of the effectiveness of alcohol education. Recommendations regarding methodological characteristics of an adequate test of effectiveness of alcohol education are presented and discussed.

186. Cooper, C., and Walker, C. (1980). Peer Dynamics final evaluation report. 1979-1980. Part 1. Lincoln, NE: Nebraska State Department of Education.

Presents the findings of Part I of the final evaluation report of a program designed to reduce risk-taking behaviors among school age youth. This program trains and supervises students who participate in a group interactions plan with other students to develop self-esteem and better communication skills. Findings include recommendations related to staff structures, time frames, and grade levels noted as appropriate for such a program.

187. Cooper, C., and Walker, C. (1980). Peer Dynamics final evaluation report. 1979-1980. Part 2. Lincoln, NE: Nebraska State Department of Education.

The findings of the second part of the final evaluation report suggests that there has been a positive attitude change among group members due to their participation in the Peer Dynamics program.

188. Coordinating Council on Juvenile Justice. (1982). Facilitation of school related approaches to delinquency prevention. Washington, DC: Author.

Presents objectives, activities, and outcomes or products of a series of steps for delinquency prevention. Suggests school related alcohol and drug abuse prevention programs, treatment alternative for alcohol and drug abusing juveniles, community activities, etc., for consideration as part of school-based programs for youth.

189. Cretcher, D. (1982). Steering clear: Helping your child through the high risk drug years. Minneapolis, MN: Winston Press.

Presents an overview of the prevalence and development of drug problems among youth. Includes information for parents and adults on how they can prevent many of these problems.

190. Cuenot, R. (1982). Evaluation of effectiveness of a one-time alcohol abuse prevention education assembly. Psychological reports, 51(2), 440-442.

Assessed prevention education measures on personal, peer, and parental behavior as viewed by 332 seventh graders in a post-test only evaluation. There were no significant findings.

191. Davis, J., Mermelstein, V., and Whitfield, C. (1982, April). Risk reduction demonstration project for adolescent alcohol use and smoking in an inner city population in Baltimore City, Maryland. Paper presented at the National Council on Alcoholism Forum, Washington, DC.

Describes a project of adolescent risk reduction for alcohol use and smoking in an inner city area where alcohol, drugs, and smoking are common among youth.

* Dembo, R., and others. (1976). Drug abuse prevention: The awareness, experience, and opinions of Junior and Senior High School students in New York State. Report No. 2 of Winter 1974-75 Survey. New York: N.Y.S. Office of Drug Abuse Services.

See No. 5.

192. Dembo, R., and Miran, M. (1975). Evaluation of drug prevention programs by youth in a middle class community. International journal of the addictions, 11(5).

Examines young peoples' reactions to various prevention programs and indicates program topics they would like to see included in future prevention efforts.

193. Des Jarlais, D., Langrod, J., Ruiz, P., and Lowinson, J. (1981). Prevention strategies in the field of substance abuse. In: J. Lowinson, and P. Ruiz (Eds.), Substance abuse: Clinical problems and perpectives. Baltimore, MD: Williams and Wilkins.

Discusses findings from a survey of high school students regarding their alcohol consumption, attitudes towards alcohol, etc. It was found that the prevalence of alcohol use in this population has risen since 1975. These data are used to substantiate the need for prevention programs.

194. DeSoto Public Schools. (1973). Drug abuse prevention education: Interim evaluation report, July 1, 1972 to June 30, 1973. DeSoto, MO: Author.

Reports the success of a drug abuse education project after one year of implementation. Progress is noted in the following areas: met instructional and educational needs;

developed and implemented a plan whereby the school worked with community, civic, religious, and fraternal organizatons; developed written procedures, teaching methods, curriculum, and materials; developed and implemented an adult-level program to disseminate factual information on the subject. The program was disseminated through intra-district communication, media, project presentations, and through other agencies.

195. Dickinson, L., and others. (1973). A comparison of three community drug abuse programs including clientele, cost, and effectiveness. Journal of drug education, 3(3), 247-259.

Compares demographic characteristics of members enrolled in three community-based treatment programs. Findings conclude that younger and unemployed clients are seen more often in Therapeutic Communities while older persons tend to be members of outpatient Methadone Maintenance Treatment Programs.

196. Domino, G. (1982). "Get high on yourself": The effectiveness of a television campaign on self-esteem, drug use, and drug attitudes. Journal of drug education, 12(2), 163-171.

Examines the effects of a three-week television campaign against drug abuse. Measurements of self-esteem, drug use, and drug attitudes were taken. Findings indicate that no significant changes could be attributed to the campaign. A significant relationship was obtained between level of self-esteem, drug use, and drug attitudes.

197. Duryea, E. (1983). Utilizing tenets of inoculation theory to develop and evaluate a preventive alcohol education intervention. Journal of school health, 53(4), 250-256.

Presents the evaluation findings of a program offered to 955 ninth graders that was based on the inoculation theory of training.

Results indicate that the formulation of prevention alcohol education programs utilizing inoculation theory in a school setting was both feasible and productive in achieving designated objectives.

198. Dusewicz, R., and Martin, M. (1981). Impacts of a Georgia drug abuse prevention program, Final Evaluation report. Philadelphia, PA: Research for Better Schools, Inc.

Presents the findings of a comprehensive evaluation of Georgia Life Skills for Mental Health and Mental Retardation, Georgia Department of Human Resources. Although the sections of the program that address teacher training were well rated, the findings were not as successful with regard to clients.

199. Education Commission of the States. (1974). Task Force on Responsible decisions about alcohol, Interim Report Number 1. Summary, technical document, and reports on working conferences. Denver, CO: Author.

Reviews the activites of the task force developed to begin a program to involve the total education system in seeking solutions to alcoholism.

200. Education Developmental Center, Inc. (1982). Protecting oneself and others: Smoking, drinking, and drugs. Newton, MA: Author.

Presents a module for prevention education contained within a health education curriculum program, TMTH Program. The goal of the program is to provide secondary school students with knowledge, skills, and an understanding that will enable them to act on behalf of themselves and others in a health-enhancing way.

201. Eiseman, S. (1971). Education about narcotics and dangerous drugs: A challenge to our schools. Journal of drug education, 1(2), 177-185.

Describes the problem of drug abuse in the schools and the role of the school as a preventive agent or deterrent. The author describes practical health education classes that may be useful in lessening this problem.

202. Emrich, R., and Green, P. (1981). Summary of the evaluation of the Phoenix Pilot Drug Program. Napa, CA: Pacific Institute for Research and Evaluation.

Summarizes the evaluation of a program whose goals are described as the development of an educational environment that will enable students to reduce their drug/alcohol usage and function in a regular school program. It focused on the relationship between parents and the school, as well as the effect and role the academic environment can play in prevention efforts.

203. European Youth Center. (1981, April). European youth center study session: "Preventive measure on alcohol and drug abuse taken or initiated by youth organizations." Conference Proceedings. Strasbourg, France.

Presents a report that reviews various aspects of the preventive measures taken by youth organizations throughout Europe. Specific strategies are described, as well as their success or failure being described.

204. Fagerberg, S., and Fagerberg, K. (1976). Student attitudes concerning drug abuse education and prevention. Journal of drug education, 6(2), 141-151.

Presents the findings of a study that surveyed the patterns of drug abuse in three academic settings. Specific recommendations and considerations to minimize drug abuse are given.

205. Flay, B., and Phil, D. (1983). Role of mass media in preventing adolescent substance abuse. NIDA research monograph no. 47: RAUS review report. Rockville, MD: National Institute on Drug Abuse.

Describes the successes and failures of various media-based drug and alcohol campaigns.

206. Fontan, M. (1983, August). Principles of prevention. In: Proceedings of the Fourth World Congress for the Prevention of Alcoholism and Drug Dependency. Nairobi, Kenya: Author.

Describes several points that have been discussed in the formulation of an alcohol abuse prevention model for youth. Defines youth at risk, prevention, and other terms related to the overall development of prevention programs.

207. Fontana, V. (1980). Child abuse: Prevention in teenage parents. New York State journal of medicine, 80(1), 53-56.

Describes the role that teenage alcoholism plays in adolescent pregnancy and describes alcoholism as one of the primary causes of child abuse.

208. Forslund, M. (1974). Indian and non-Indian delinquency: A self report study of Wind River Reservation area youth. Washington, DC: Youth Development and Delinquency Prevention Administration.

Describes a study that examined the drug use patterns and attitudes towards drugs between Indian youth and non-Indian youth in Wyoming. It is noted that there is little difference between these groups, with the exception of Indian youth having more problems centered around the school and having used more drugs other than marijuana.

209. French, J. (Ed.). (1983). Working with evaluators: A guide for drug abuse prevention program managers. Trenton, NJ: New Jersey State Department of Health.

Introduces the conceptual framework for an evaluation model as part of a nine-step continual process of program planning, feedback, and change. Delineates issues of prevention evaluation discussed from the program manager's perspective.

210. Frenkel, S., and others. (1974). Drug use: Demography and attitudes in a Junior and Senior High School population. Journal of drug education, 4(2), 179-186.

Describes a survey that was undertaken to provide descriptive information and correlational data related to drug use in junior and senior high school populations to assist in the development, planning, and evaluation of prevention services.

211. Fried, J., and Cimaglio, R. (1983, April). Market research approach to prevention. Paper presented at the National Council on Alcoholism Forum, Houston, TX.

Describes the approach to prevention developed by the Illinois Council on Alcoholism. This program has developed two pevention campaigns which address community needs from primary to tertiary prevention efforts.

212. Gallant, D. (1983). Adolescent drinking: The road toward prevention. Alcoholism: Clinical and experimental research, 7(1), 100.

Describes the results of a survey that studied self-concept, alcohol education, and drinking habits. The author contends that knowledge about alcohol alone does not have any effect on reduction of drinking. Further, the author questions the value of education prevention programs that fail to use personality antecedents to alcohol use. Recommendations are made for protocols to be developed as part of prevention efforts.

213. Geis, G., and others. (1969). Ex-addicts as streetworkers. The Boyle Heights Narcotics Prevention Project. Los Angeles, CA: California State College.

Discusses what the project was designed to achieve, what is accomplished, and how. The strengths and weaknesses of the program are indicated. The report concludes that, based on the numbers of persons serviced, the project was seen as a needed and appreciated service.

214. General Research Corp. (1973). Case studies of selected components of the Office of Education community drug abuse prevention projects. Volume I. Executive summary. Washington, DC: Department of Health, Education and Welfare.

Presents ten case studies to evaluate the effectiveness of community drug abuse prevention programs. Identifies strengths and weaknesses of individual projects with generalization to other prevention efforts.

215. General Research Corp. (1973). Case studies of selected components of the Office of Education community drug abuse prevention projects. Volume II. Study methodology and findings. Washington, DC: Department of Health, Education and Welfare.

Presents a study whose objective was to provide the Office of the Assistant Secretary for Planning of the Office of Education with information relative to the operation and effectiveness of the Office of Education's prevention programs. Presented in the fashion of case studies with supporting data.

216. General Research Corp. (1973). Evaluation of selected components of the Office of Education "Help Communities Help Themselves" drug abuse prevention program. Washington, DC: Department of Health, Education and Welfare.

Presents the Help Communities Help Themselves drug abuse prevention program and the evaluation of this project. The goal of the program was to assist communities mobilize their own resources and develop prevention efforts that reflect their immediate needs.

217. General Research Corp. (1973). Evaluation of selected components of the Office of Education "Help Communities Help Themselves" drug abuse prevention program, Volume I: Executive Summary. Washington, DC: Department of Health, Education and Welfare.

Describes a program developed to train communities in the development of prevention programs that will best meet their needs. The principal purpose of this evaluation was to determine the effectiveness of the HCHT Training Program.

218. General Research Corp. (1973). Evaluation of selected components of the Office of Education "Help Communities Help Themselves" drug abuse prevention program, Volume II: Evaluation methodology and findings. Washington, DC: Department of Health, Education and Welfare.

Describes the evaluation methodology and findings of the evaluation of the HCHT program. The approach was to have investigators visit and conduct field studies in respective communities that had participated in the HCHT program. Data related to the effectiveness of this project are presented.

219. General Research Corp. (1973). Evaluation of selected components of the Office of Education "Help Communities Help Themselves": Drug abuse prevention program, Volume III: Questionnaires. Washington, DC: Department of Health, Education and Welfare.

Presents the findings of an evaluation that attempted to evaluate the effectiveness of the HCHT Training Program where effectiveness was determined in terms of activity levels resulting from the training process.

220. Gilmin, H. (Ed.). (1982). Youth problems. Washington, DC: Congressional Quarterly.

Presents editorial research on youth problems. Specific reports discuss drug abuse and alcohol abuse, while other reports address topics such as suicide, juvenile justice, violence in the family, etc. Specific attention is placed on the need to develop viable prevention efforts and programs. Suggestions for consideration are made.

221. Gilson, S. (Ed.). (1981). Steven Glenn on prevention. Lincoln, NE: University of Nebraska.

Summarizes the comments at a seminar on drug and alcohol prevention. Recommendations for areas to be considered in the development and evaluation of prevention programs are made.

222. Globetti, G. (1983). General considerations on prevention of alcohol abuse and alcohol problems in children and adolescents. In: O. Jeanneret (Ed.), Alcohol and youth. Basel, Switzerland: S. Karger.

Describes four models of prevention programs. These span programs from those that view the drug itself as being the source, to those that believe that drinking in concert with vulnerable personalities leads to problems. Consideration is given to what research suggests about prevention activities for youth.

* Gluckstern, N. (1973). Training parents as drug counselors in the community. Personnel and Guidance Journal, 51, 676-680.

See No. 574.

223. Goodstadt, M., Sheppard, M., and Chan, G. (1981). An evaluation model of two school based alcohol education programs. Toronto, Canada: Addiction Research Foundation.

Reviews prior evaluation models of alcohol education prevention programs and 21 alcoholism prevention programs; suggestions for a model evaluation program for school based programs are made.

224. Greenwell, G. (1980). Counseling for alcohol, tobacco, and drug abuse. Searchlight Plus: Relevant Resources in High Interest Areas, 50.

Reviews the literature on counseling for alcohol, tobacco and drug abuse. The introduction highlights specific issues and trends in drug abuse prevention programs at the elementary, junior high, high school, college and community levels.

225. Griffin, T. (1983). Role of activity director and coach in response to student chemical use problems. Anoka, MN: Minnesota High School League.

Discusses the role of coaches, activity directors, teachers, counselors, and administrators in the prevention of substance abuse through influencing student behaviors with proper drug education curriculum and instruction.

226. Gunther, E. (1980, November). Evaluation of drug misuse prevention. Paper presented at the workshop on "Aspects of aid to drug addicts," Hamburg, W. Germany, Hamburg Health Authority.

Discusses the problems of legal and illegal drug use, etiology of drug misuse, and presents a four step plan for influencing human behavior with respect to drug misuse.

227. Gyllander, N. (1983, April). Preventive programs for youth. Paper presented at the National Council on Alcoholism Forum, Houston, TX.

Describes a model drug abuse prevention program for rural communities. This program included a leadership camp, a teen institute, and school awareness days. The objective is for youth to become more aware of themselves and their relationships with others, and that, consequently, this would have an effect on drug abuse. The author notes that the program was successful in meeting its stated goals.

228. Haenn, J. (1984). Evaluation of Project HAPPIER Survey: Illinios. Harrisburg, PA: Pennsylvania State Department of Education.

Presents the findings of a survey conducted among teachers and migrant personnel in Illinois to assess the current health needs of migrants. The availability of educational materials was also investigated in order to ensure that a proposed health resource guide would meet the needs of migrant health and educational staff and parents. Dental health, nutrition, fitness, and substance abuse were listed as the most serious concerns.

229. Hamburg, D., Elliot, G., and Parron, D. (1982). Health and behavior: Frontiers of research in the biobehavioral sciences. Washington, DC: National Academy Press.

Describes findings from research efforts that focused on alcohol abuse. Efforts to prevent alcohol abuse among adolescents are described.

230. Hanson, D. (1982). The effectiveness of alcohol and drug education. Journal of alcohol and drug education, 27(2), 1-13.

Examines articles that have evaluated prevention efforts. Organizes these into separate categories; those that have investigated drug knowledge; those that have investigated drug attitudes; those that have considered both knowledge and attitudes; and those that have explored drug use.

231. Harrison-Burns, B., and others. (1981). A guide to multicultural drug abuse prevention: Evaluation series handbook. Rockville, MD: National Institute on Drug Abuse.

Addresses several issues related to program evaluation for prevention programs designed for minority populations. These issues included planning, the role of the evaluator, selection of the evaluation methodology, selection of data collection instruments, training of data collection staff, analysis of data, reporting the findings, and use of the evaluation results for program improvement.

232. Harten, R. (1982). Normal and addicted: Addiction in our society, materials for prevention. Kiel, W. Germany: Aktion Jugendschutz.

Published originally in German, presents various problems of addiction. Prevention efforts are reviewed and discussed.

233. Hedin, D., and Norem-Hebeisen, A. (1983). Influences on adolescent problem behavior: Causes, connections, and contexts. In: R. Isralowitz, and M. Singer (Eds.). Adolescent; A guide to prevention and treatment. New York, NY: Haworth Press.

Describes conceptual and empirical evidence for correlates of problem behavior in general. Drug and alcohol abuse, in particular, are examined, emphasizing that peer influence can be an effective means of preventing drug abuse.

234. Hewitt, K. (1976). The whole college catalog about drinking: A guide to alcohol abuse prevention. Rockville, MD: National Institute on Alcohol Abuse and Alcoholism.

Attempts to encourage new thinking about alcohol use and abuse. It presents a comprehensive and useful approach to alcohol abuse prevention. Each section is a separate unit that can be used independently of the remaining sections to address distinct topics. Helpful in developing new approaches to alcohol abuse on the campus. Describes ways to develop, evaluate, and monitor school based prevention programs.

235. Homel, R. (1982, April). Deterring the drinking driver: Should young drivers be the target? Paper presented at the Seminar on the Place of the Driver in Road Safety, Newcastle, Australia.

Examines the effectiveness of the procedures currently used by police and the courts to deal with young drinking and driving offenders in Australia. Presents statistics relative to this.

236. Horan, J., and others. (1975). Behavioral counseling: Training and treatment research at the Pennsylvania State University. Washington, DC: American Educational Research Association.

Presents brief reports on the empirical findings that have emerged from many sources on the subject of behavioral counseling. Two distinct strands are noted; the first is the training process whereby specifics are taught, the second category speaks to assertion training, decision training, emotive imagery, etc. No comments are made on the relevancy or superiority of either strand.

* Horan, J., and others. (1973). A training model for drug abuse prevention: Content and evaluation. Journal of drug education, 3(2), 121-126.

See No. 37.

237. Horan, J., and Williams, J. (1975). The tentative drug use scale: A quick and relatively problem free outcome measure for drug abuse prevention projects. Journal of drug education. 5(4), 381-384.

Describes the Tentative Drug Use Scale, an instrument designed to assist in obtaining behavioral data. Advantages of this scale over others are discussed. Reliability and validity data are provided.

238. Hu, T., and Swisher, J. (1983). Alternatives to drug abuse: Some are and some are not. In: Preventing adolescent drug abuse: Intervention strategies. Rockville, MD: National Institute on Drug Abuse.

Describes several prevention efforts and indicates that many of these do not prevent the abuse of drugs, in fact, some may even encourage such abuse.

239. Jessor, R., and Perry, C. (1983). Doing the cube: Preventing drug abuse through adolescent health promotion. NIDA research monograph no. 47: RAUS review report. Rockville, MD: National Institute on Drug Abuse.

Describes the role of health promotion as an intervention modality. Presents a four-pronged approach to health including: physical health; psychological health; social health; personal health. The authors conclude that through this approach smoking, drinking and marijuana use can be curtailed.

240. Johnson, D. (1975, March-April). Cooperative competencies and the prevention and treatment of drug abuse. Paper presented at the Annual Meeting of the American Educational Research Association, Washington, DC.

Describes the competencies required in individuals who are least likely to use drugs and further describes the development of these competencies as a model for prevention efforts.

241. Johnson, N. (1982). Michigan develops curriculum to reduce DWI among youth. Alcohol, health and research world, 7(1), 35-37.

Describes the development, implementation, and evaluation of an education program designed to reduce DWI's through a curriculum-bound alcohol abuse prevention program. The program is comprised of four curriculum modules. The data indicate that results were successful and retained by students for at least several months.

242. Jones, R. (1984). Navy substance abuse prevention program: Research and evaluation. Paper presented at the Annual Convention of the American Psychological Association, Toronto, Canada.

The importance and usefulness of the formative and summative evaluations are discussed and specific evaluation tasks are identified. These include personnel selection and the functions and qualifications of various personnel. It further describes the intervention process and personnel training. Other areas include curriculum, classroom management, and participant characteristics.

243. Judd, G. (1982). Testimony for the Senate Alcoholism and Drug Abuse Subcommittee. In: Hearing . . . Ninety-seventh Congress. Salt Lake City, UT: Utah Congress of Parents and Teachers.

Presents the concerns of the Utah State Congress of Parents and Teachers as they relate to drug prevention. Recommendations for Federal response to prevention efforts are made.

244. Kakalik, J., and others. (1976). Mental health and mental retardation services in Nevada, executive summary. Reno, NV: Max C. Fleischmann Foundation.

Summarizes the findings and recommendations of a two-year study of all major services and service delivery systems in Nevada for persons with mental health disorders, mentally retarded persons, and abusers of alcohol and drugs. Addresses special area needs and concludes with 71 specific recommendations for services and the delivery system.

245. Kassebaum, P., Hathaway, B., and Mong, M. (1981). On the sidelines: An adult leader guide for youth alcohol programs. Rockville, MD: NIAAA, National Clearinghouse for Alcohol Information.

Describes activities, materials, etc., for professionals and others who have never worked in an alcohol program for youth. Designed to stimulate and support lively alcohol abuse prevention projects conducted by youth, for youth, on issues that interest and affect them.

246. Kearney, A., and Hines, M. (1980). Evaluation of the effectiveness of a drug prevention education program. Journal of drug education, 10(2), 127-134.

Presents the evaluation of the Cooperative Educational Service Agency No. Eight in Wisconsin. As a result of this evaluation, the program won recognition from the U.S. Office of Education as a national model program.

247. Kentucky Department of Education, Bureau of Instruction. (1980). Making decisions: Alcohol and drug education guide K-12. Frankfort, KY: Author.

Describes drug prevention efforts that can be used in the classroom. Uses a three-pronged approach to drug education to enable students to: (1) increase their knowledge about drugs; (2) develop skills in making decisions about drugs; (3) clarify their values regarding drug use.

248. Kern, J. (1974). Evaluating community drug abuse agencies. Journal of drug education, 4(2), 129-139.

Reviews the lack of evaluations in the literature that addresses storefront drug treatment prevention agencies. Suggestions are given for a five-step procedure for such evaluations and reviews.

249. Kim, S. (1982). An approach toward quality control of workshops. Journal of drug education, 12(1), 55-63.

Introduces a practical approach toward the quality control of workshops given in the field of drug abuse prevention and in community mental health settings. Describes the workshop questionnaire which probes respondents' overall reaction, workshop effectiveness, and application of techniques to participants' environments.

250. Kim, S. (1981). An evaluation of Ombudsman Primary Prevention Program on student drug abuse. Journal of drug education, 11(1), 27-636.

Presents the findings of the program evaluation of a prevention program that had as its aim to elicit positive changes in "high risk" attitudinal states of students. Results indicated favorably attitudinal changes by participants towards teachers, OP trained instructors, and teachers. The program was more effective with elementary students.

251. Kim, S. (1982). Feeder area approach: An impact evaluation of a prevention project on student drug abuse. International journal of the addictions, 17(2), 305-313.

Investigated the effect of a community-based prevention program by implementing a feeder area approach over a two-year period. A significant reduction had been found in the area of the county where this service had been offered as compared to the pre-test results.

252. Kim, S. (1981). How do we know whether a primary prevention program on drug abuse works or does not work? International journal of the addictions, 16(2), 359-365.

Presents a program evaluation of the Ombudsman Program, a primary prevention program developed by the Charlotte Drug Education Center. Findings indicate that the program is most effective with hard drugs but not as effective with social drugs, the program impacts young students more successfully.

253. Kim, S. (1982). A uniform progress and evaluation reporting system for alcohol and drug abuse prevention agencies: Two examples. Journal of drug education, 12(4), 309-323.

Provides a systematic approach toward a remedy of the stagnation in program monitoring and program evaluation for the fields of prevention and intervention.

254. Kim, S., Hoffman, I., Pike, M., and Gibson, J. (1984). An outcome evaluation instrument for alcohol education, prevention and intervention programs. Journal of drug education, 14(4), 331-346.

Introduces the Alcohol Education Evaluation Instrument, a theoretically-based tool for outcome evaluation of the effectiveness of alcohol education, prevention, and intervention programs designed to deter adolescent alcohol abuse. The instrument is reported to measure behavioral, intentional, attitudinal, and informational changes in the subject.

255. Kinard, B. (1982). 97th Congress, February 1982, Testimony of Beverly J. Kinard. In: Hearing ... Ninety-Seventh Congress. Salt Lake City, UT: Utah Congress of Parents and Teachers.

Presents the testimony of a parent before a U.S. Senate Committee on how her son became involved in drugs, briefly discusses the role and responsibilities of parents, teachers, and the federal government in the prevention of drug abuse. Resource materials and curriculum on prevention programs are provided.

256. Kinsey, B., and others. (1975). A comparative study of non-opiate and clinical patients: Implications for education and prevention. Journal of drug education, 5(2), 141-150.

Presents a study that examines the appropriateness of the preventive mental health model of prevention by comparing a group of non-opiate drug abusers with a psychiatric group. Findings indicate that both groups share similarities. The authors indicate that non-opiate abusers showed more psychosocial adjustment problems than other clinical patients.

257. Klee, T. (1983). Effectiveness of a model drug and alcohol abuse prevention program on low risk students. Dissertation abstracts international, 44(3), 710-A.

Presents the results of an evaluation of prevention services in ten Philadephia high schools. Findings suggest that a positive impact was realized with variation by school. Suggests reasons for these variations.

258. Kleinman, S., and Olsen, L. (1973). An evaluation of the long range effects of drug education workshops. Journal of school health, 43(9), 578-583.

Presents an evaluation of the effects of drug education workshops. Findings reveal that time was not a decisive factor in subsequent drug education activities, and that training programs are ineffectual in stimulating attitude change.

259. Kleinot, M., and Rogers, R. (1982). Identifying effective components of alcohol misuse prevention programs. Journal of studies on alcohol, 43(7), 802-811.

Reports the findings of a study that shows the effectiveness of three components of many programs for the prevention of alcohol misuse and alcoholism: the severity of the consequences of excessive drinking, an individual's personal vulnerability to these unpleasant consequences, and the effectiveness of moderate or responsible drinking in preventing these problems.

260. Koberl, I. (1981). Thoughts on drug prevention and prophylaxis. Wiener zeitschrift fuer such forschung, 4(1), 17-19.

Presents probable psychosocial causes of addictive behavior and their prevention. The author indicates that the most powerful influences on drug use are parent and peer pressure and that, therefore, prevention efforts should attempt to gain the support of parents and peer influences. It is noted that these groups should look to raise the individual's awareness of social pressures and responsibilities.

261. Kohn, P., Goodstadt, M., Cook, G., Sheppard, M., and Chan, G. (1982). Ineffectiveness of threat appeals about drinking and driving. Accident analysis and prevention, 14(6), 457-464.

Presents data from a study where students were exposed to films designed to elicit varying degrees of general upset. It was discovered that the films that elicited feelings of threat, as opposed to just fear, outscored the control groups' results.

262. Konigsberg, D., Weinhouse, B., and Wechsler, J. (1983). Teenagers and alcohol: Holiday hazard, year round tragedy. Ladies home journal, 100(12), 78, 80, 86-87.

Presents statistics on and examples of the tragedies caused by teenaged drinking. These statistics are used to illustrate the nature and extent of the alcohol problem and youth.

263. Kraft, D. (1979). Public drinking practices of college youths: Implications for prevention programs. In: T.C. Harford and L.S. Gaines (Eds.), Social drinking contexts. Monograph No. 7. Washington, DC: National Institute on Drug Abuse.

Describes the drinking behaviors and attitudes of college students. Provides approaches for prevention efforts on campus. These include both direct and indirect approaches.

264. Kramer, R. (1982). Statement by Robert G. Kramer. In: Hearing ... Ninety-Seventh Congress. Washington, DC: United States Government Printing Office.

Presents the prevention efforts of the Anne Arundel County Drug and Alcohol Program.

265. Krokfore, K. (1979). Preventive action in the field of alcohol policy. In P. Duda et al. (Eds.), Alcohol and youth. Warsaw, Poland: Psychoneurological Institute.

Outlines the policy of the Ministry of Social Affairs and Health of Finland. Many of the activities include education to develop positive attitudes towards drug and alcohol abuse.

266. Lambert, C. (1983). Teenage alcohol and smoking prevalence data. In: Report of the Health Education Risk Reduction Conference. Anaheim, CA: October 1981.

Presents prevalence data from smoking and alcohol intervention projects in Massachusetts. The data are useful to target intervention programs to the students at risk, assist educators in developing prevention programs in schools, and assists in developing more appropriate modeling for adults.

* Larsen, B., Krynak, D., and Pettyjohn, T. (1981). Alcohol and other drug use among rural adolescents: Some implications for rural drug programming. In: A.J. Schecter (Ed.), Drug dependency and alcoholism, Vol. 2: Social behavior issues. New York, NY: Plenum Press.

See No. 109.

267. Lerner, S., and Linder, R. (1974). Drugs in the elementary school. Journal of drug education, 4(3), 317-322.

Describes a study used to determine at what grade levels and to what extent upper elementary school students initiate use of psychoactive drugs, reasons for use, and availability of drugs within the school.

268. Lipinska-Broja, W. (1979). Program of preventive activity of the National Committee among the school youth. In: P. Duda et al. (Eds.), Alcohol and youth. Warsaw, Poland: Psychoneurological Institute.

Describes a civic organization that initiated and coordinated activities designed to inform and organize the public for the fight against alcoholism in Warsaw.

269. Lipton, W. (1977, June). Alcohol handicapped child. Paper presented at the 23rd International Institute on Prevention and Treatment of Alcoholism, Dresden, Germany.

Presents the results of various studies conducted in Yugoslavia, Austria, and West Germany to demonstrate the social degradation of children in alcoholic families, and the negative physical, mental, and spiritual effects of parental alcoholism. Preventive measures for children of alcoholic families are outlined.

270. Little, Arthur, Inc. (1974). Evaluation of services offered by community mental health centers (CMHCs) and ADAMHA funded drug and alcohol programs to juvenile delinquents: Volume I. Rockville, MD: National Institute of Mental Health.

Presents findings related to the determination of the nature, extent, and interrelationships of services offered by CMHCs and ADAMHA funded community based drug and alcohol programs to juvenile delinquents in order to help determine the appropriate role of health agencies in serving juvenile delinquents within the community.

271. Lopez, T., and Starkey, K. (1976). A primary prevention drug education program for school children: An attempt at evaluation. Paper presented at the Annual Meeting of the American Educational Research Association. San Francisco, CA.

Presents the findings of an evaluation of drug prevention services that used an affective education model. Findings conclude that children grew in self-esteem and had a more positive attitude toward risk taking; although value sharing activities did not increase after teacher training was completed.

272. Lotecka, L. (1974). A project advocating humanistic education: An evaluation of its effects on public school teachers. Journal of drug education, 4(2), 141-149.

An evaluation of a seminar on preventing drug abuse shows that participating classroom teachers gained significantly in drug knowledge. There were also significant changes in attitudes concerning drug abuse, child development, and pedagogy.

273. Lowman, C. (1983, April). Implication of national data for the development of alcohol countermeasures. Paper presented at the Lifesaver II Panel Conference, Denver, CO.

Presents data on the prevalence and nature of teenage drinking. The author concludes that to achieve long term success in preventing teenage alcohol use, it will be particularly important to develop strategies that are self-renewing at the grass roots level.

* Lynch, M. (1967). "US": Primary prevention, paracounseling, research project. Rockville, MD: National Institute on Drug Abuse.

See No. 111.

274. Maine Office of Alcoholism and Drug Abuse Prevention. (1976). Five-year forward plan for comprehensive alcoholism services for Maine. Augusta, ME: Author.

Describes the plan for approaching the drug abuse and alcoholism needs for the state of Maine. The plan includes types, volume, cost, and benefits of needed prevention, treatment, and rehabilitative services. Also included are issues of training, evaluation of services, needs assessments, and legislative assistance. Indicates the year-by-year implementation of proposed programs.

275. Malvin, J., and others. (1985). Evaluation of two school-based alternatives programs.

<u>Journal of alcohol and drug education</u>, <u>30</u>(3), 98-108.

Reports the results of two evaluations of school-based service opportunity programs for junior high school students. Collects affective and drug-specific measures and hypothesizes towards effects for self-esteem, attitudes toward school, attendance, and locus of control.

276. Marion, D. (1973). <u>Crisis intervention project, Boston Public Schools, Dec. 1, 1972-May 1, 1973, Evaluation</u>. Boston, MA: Data Education, Inc.

Includes two parts: the first a six-month evaluation report and the second, an interim report by the project director. Training programs, specific problems of the project, initial impact areas, and related projects are discussed. Results of brief needs assessment survey of staff and board members are included.

277. Martin, G., Ward, E. and Newmas, I. (1982). <u>Evaluation as a part of primary prevention programming: The Indian Youth Project</u>. Lincoln, NE: University of Nebraska, Nebraska Center for Alcohol and Drug Abuse.

Describes the efforts that were made to increase the specificity and usefulness of evaluating a primary prevention program. It has the objective improvement of interpersonal skills and abilities among its participants. The report concludes with an outline of psychosocial development to be monitored, a training manual developed for the staff of the center for behavior documentation, and a behavior documentation chart.

278. Mason, V. and Baker, G. (1978). <u>Growing up and feeling powerful as an American Indian</u>. Rockville, MD: National Institute of Drug Abuse.

Presents a program prepared for American

Indian school children in grades 4-8. Materials and curriculum are based on primary prevention concepts, created by Native American experts involved in various aspects in drug abuse treatment. Materials are presented in a cultural context based on Native American cultural values and belief systems.

279. Messolonghites, L. (1976). Primary prevention in drug abuse: An annotated guide to the literature. Rockville, MD: National Institute on Drug Abuse.

Presents an annotated guide to literature relevant to primary prevention. Includes areas of history, strategies, policies on drug abuse prevention, education and training, community action, multimedia information sources, evaluations, and State and Federal contacts and coordinators.

280. Michigan State Department of Education. (1975). Substance abuse prevention education program. 1974-75 Evaluation report. Lansing, MI: Author.

Describes the multi-faceted aims and goals of this prevention program, as well as the activities that were conducted during the year of 1974-75. Materials are presented that may be of use to evaluators working with other projects.

281. Millman, R., and Khuri, E. (1981). Adolescence and substance abuse. In: J.H. Lowinson, and P. Ruiz (Eds.), Substance abuse: Clinical problems and perspectives. Baltimore, MD: Williams and Wilkins.

Discusses adolescent substance abuse under the following topics: (1) patterns of use and abuse; (2) epidemiology; (3) determinants of abuse behavior; and (4) prevention and treatment.

282. Millman, R. and Khuri, E. (1982). Alcohol and adolescent psychopathology.

In: J. Solomon (Ed.), Alcoholism and clinical psychiatry. New York, NY: Plenum Medical Book.

Cites literature in a discussion of alcohol and adolescent psychopathology. Addresses the following issues: patterns of usage; determinants of abusive behavior; prevention and treatment approaches.

283. Mills, K., Neal, E., and Peed-Neal, I. (1983). Handbook for alcohol education: The community approach. Cambridge, MA: Ballinger.

Presents an education handbook intended for use in higher education institutions. The first part addresses the community systems model and how to coordinate training curriculum for program personnel. The second part addresses self-instruction modules for peer educators.

284. Monroe-Scott, B., and Miranda, V. (1981). Guidebook for planning alcohol prevention programs with black youth. Rockville, MD: NIAAA, Clearinghouse for Alcohol Information.

Presents ideas for program development for services targeted at black youth. The authors suggest steps for program implementation using an inter-agency network approach.

* Morriss, R. (1983). Peer education teaches Minnesota teenagers the control factor in drinking and driving. Traffic safety, 83(5), 6-8.

See No. 116.

285. Morton, Anton, et al. (1973, October). An evaluation of drug education in the United States Army. Paper presented at the International Council on Drug Education.

Presents data on the drug education prevention program developed by the armed forces for enlisted men. The findings indicate that there was little effect of the prevention effort but the authors conclude that the impact might have been different had the audience consisted of younger school children who had not yet tried drugs. Reasons for the failure of the project are given.

* Moser, J. (1980). Prevention of alcohol related problems. Toronto, Canada: Addiction Research Foundation Marketing Services.

See No. 117.

286. Moskowitz, J. (1983). Preventing adolescent substance abuse through drug education. In: Preventing adolescent drug abuse: Intervention strategies. Rockville, MD: National Institute on Drug Abuse.

Examines the efficacy of drug education as a prevention solution to substance abuse. Discusses the three most common models of prevention efforts; knowledge/attitude approach, values/decision making approach, and the social competency approach. The authors indicate that there is little value to support these models.

287. Moskowitz, J. (1983). Discussion and recommendations. In: Preventing adolescent drug abuse: Intervention strategies. Rockville, MD: National Institute on Drug Abuse.

Reviews research on prevention attempts for adolescents. Discusses the goals as outlined by prevention programs. Makes recommendations for future efforts of other prevention programs.

288. Moskowitz, J., et al. (1981). A process and outcome evaluation of a peer teaching primary prevention program. Napa, CA: Pacific Institute for Research and Evaluation.

Describes an evaluation that was used to determine the effectiveness of Jigsaw, a structured peer teaching program in which students teach part of the regular classroom curriculum to a group of peers. The goal was to make students play a more active role in the learning process. It is the belief of the authors that this type of learning activity makes it less likely that involved students will use illicit drugs or alcohol.

289. Moskowitz, J., Malvin, J. Schaeffer, G., and Schaps, E. (1983). Evaluation of a junior high school primary prevention program. Addictive behaviors, 8(4), 393-401.

Presents the results of a two-year evaluation of a prevention program offered in a junior high school. Although positive effects were found for females on several drug related variables, few effects were found for males. Individual prevention strategies are presented.

290. Moskowitz, J., Schaps, E., Schaeffer, G., and Malvin, J. (1984). Evaluation of a substance abuse prevention program for junior high school students. International journal of the addictions, 19(4), 419-430.

Discusses the effects of two prevention strategies offered in junior high schools. One junior high school was offered in-service training for teaching staff, affective Classroom Management Training, with all seventh grade students receiving drug education; the other school received neither of these. Results indicate that drug education holds some promise as a substance abuse preventive measure. The findings are not clear on the effects of in-service teacher training.

291. Murrell, W. (1979). A study of multi-cultural alternatives to drug abuse in New Mexico. Boulder, CO: Resources Development Internship Program.

Describes an evaluation of five drug abuse prevention programs in New Mexico that offered services to Indians and Mexicans. The purpose was to determine which elements were successful in meeting their goals. Results indicated that the ability to communicate meaningfully with ethnic participants in alternative prevention actitivies may depend on the prevention staff's ability to understand the mental and physical circumstances specific to their ethnic target population, which contribute to dependencies on chemical substances. This study also indicated that funding should be solicited from federal, state, and local levels, with emphasis on local funding to insure program longevity. The author notes that a needs assessment of the community is essential, that goals and objectives must reflect the immediate community, that community awareness and support is essential, and that the program's success will depend on its ability to meet community needs.

292. Nash, G. (1973). The impact of drug abuse treatment upon criminality: A look at 19 programs. Upper Montclair, NJ: Montclair State College.

Reports on a study of large scale treatment of drug abuse in the state of New Jersey. The report challenges traditional views about treatment and makes suggestions for more effective programming and treatment. Evaluates both methadone maintenance and drug-free treatment programs.

293. National Institute on Drug Abuse. (1974). Integrated drug abuse management information system briefing report. Rockville, MD: Author.

Reports on the evaluation developed as a result of the development of the Special Action Office for Drug Abuse Prevention. The evaluation included the extent of the drug problem among youth and to, specifically, identify programs developed to deal with this problem. Reports of the system developed to maintain the above referenced information on a national basis are presented.

294. National School Boards Association. (1980). Report of the 1979-80 task force on alcohol and drug abuse among students. Washington, DC: Author.

Presents the accomplishments of the task force on alcohol and drug abuse. Reviews school activities geared towards prevention; studies and compares the prevention programs presented at the meetings. Presents a composite prevention model for alcohol abuse education and prevention programs. Recommendations for prevention programs are made.

295. Newman, D. (1979). An approach to combat student misbehavior at the ninth grade level: The Committee on Referral and Evaluation (C.O.R.E.). Miami, FL: Nova University.

Describes the second phase of a two-phased practicum designed to improve the behaviors of students. The program combined school, community, and state agencies in an effort to intervene at an early level to solve current problems and to prevent future ones. It is noted that as a result of C.O.R.E. two other programs were developed, a drug abuse prevention program, and a career counseling program.

* Nowliss, H. (1977). Statement before the Subcommittee on Alcoholism and Drug Abuse, Committee on Human Resources, United States Senate. Washington, DC: United States Government Printing Office.

See No. 609.

296. Ohio Department of Health, Division of Alcoholism. (1983). 1983 Teenage Institute for the Prevention of Alcohol and other Drug Abuse. Columbus, OH: Author.

Presents and outlines the goals, objectives, and approaches to prevention used by the Teenage Institute for the Prevention of Alcohol and Drug Abuse. Includes a directory of alcoholism programs and resource materials available in the State of Ohio.

297. Ohio Department of Mental Health and Mental Retardation. (1976). State of Ohio performance report on drug abuse prevention plan, 1976. Columbus, OH: Author.

Presents an overview of the drug abuse problem in the State of Ohio and prevention efforts established as a response to this problem. Includes recommendations that address topics such as training, issues of treatment needs, education and prevention, manpower development, and research. Treats topics such as funding, treatment of special populations, rural area programming, services to abusers within the criminal justice system, involvement of the Community Mental Health System, and the relationship between the State and treatment providers.

298. O'Shea, P. and Hayes, W. (1982). Alcohol abuse in adolescents. Nurse practitioner, 7(8), 31-35.

Presents alcohol abuse among youth as a major primary health care problem. Discusses the various detriments of alcohol consumption among adolescents. Recommends prevention, early detection, and referral strategies.

299. Overend, R. (1982). You can say no to alcohol: Government media campaign for teens and women. Traffic safety, 8(4), 18-20.

Describes the development of a government sponsored alcohol awareness campaign, specifically targeted toward teenagers and women. Includes materials used in the campaign.

300. PACE Management Associates. (1979). A potpourri of program practices. (Report Series 42, Number 1). Washington, DC: Author.

Presents brief descriptions of program practices deemed innovative, unique, or facilitative, and potentially capable of adaptation by other state and local level program managers. Presents materials that may be useful for program staff for and about former drug abusers.

301. Palais, E. (1973). Drug abuse treatment: The cart before the horse. Journal of drug education, 3(2), 153-155.

Discusses the need for funding to be developed that will allow for the development of prevention programs. The author contends that money is focused towards treatment and rehabilitation when there continues to be a need for a focus towards prevention and a willingness for people to admit that a problem exists.

302. Parker, J. (1981). Drugs and alcohol: A handbook for young people. Phoenix, AZ: Do It Now Foundation.

Provides information on drugs and alcohol, their effects, and how they work, to help young people make decisions about drugs.

303. Payton, C. (1979, September). Multicultural approaches in alcohol, drug abuse and mental health prevention programs. Paper presented at the Annual Conference on Prevention of the Alcohol, Drug Abuse and Mental Health Administration. Silver Springs, MD.

Summarizes some of the recent research and evaluation of drug and other substance abuse prevention programs and directs attention to the work of Federal agencies. The author contends that the bulk of the research on drug abuse fails to consider those social and economic factors that require different and more complex solutions for minority drug abuse problems.

* Pearson, J. (1971). Juvenile drug abuse prevention project. First year evaluation report. Washington, DC: National Institute of Law Enforcement and Criminal Justice.

See No. 511.

304. Pegel, V. (1981, April). "How can young people be motivated for preventive work?" Paper presented at the European Youth Center Study Session, Strasbourg, France.

Outlines the motivational process for youth and describes ways to persuade young people not to get involved with drugs and alcohol.

305. Pentz, M. (1983). Prevention of adolescent substance abuse through social skill development. In: Preventing adolescent drug abuse: Intervention strategies. Rockville, MD: National Institute on Drug Abuse.

Evaluates the social skills training approach for preventing adolescent substance abuse. Suggestions for future research of this approach are presented.

306. Phelps, D. (1976, September). Issues in primary prevention in substance abuse. A statement. Paper presented at the Annual Convention of the American Psychological Association. Washington, DC.

Describes some of the issues that developers of primary prevention programs face. The author describes these as funding competition, the power of the alcohol industry, and the lack of relevant data on program effectiveness.

307. Planka-Syroka, B. (1983). Motivation of High School students for the use of stimulants. Problemy alkoholizmu, 30(5), 12-13.

Presents the findings of a survey of Polish high school students and the prevalence of substance abuse among those sampled. Recommendations for prevention programs are included.

308. Plat, P. (1981). Alcohol in the school age child. Revue de L'alcoolisme, 27(1), 31-42.

Presents the biological effects of alcohol on school children and the effects on developmental process. Education for parents is recommended as well as media campaigns targeted towards youth.

* Pringle, H., Gregory, J., Ginkel, K., and Cheek, C. (1981). Alpha centers: A viable prevention model for substance abuse agencies and public schools. In: A.J. Schecter (Ed.), Drug dependency and alcoholism, Vol. 2: Social behavior issues. New York, NY: Plenum Press.

See No. 126.

309. Raymond, A. (1983). Young drunk drivers course--A new approach in Australia. Globe, 1(17), 19.

Describes a program where the Department of Community Medicine of St. Vincent's Hospital uses drinking and driving convictions as an opportunity for intervention. A full description of the program essentials are given. It is reported that this effort has been successful.

310. Research for Better Schools, Inc. (1980). Impacts of a Georgia drug abuse prevention program: An evaluation research study of the Georgia Life Skills for Mental Health Program. Second Annual Report. Philadelphia, PA: Author.

Describes the evaluation report of a program that is designed as a primary prevention program which utilizes community mental health agencies as the link between program sponsors and public schools.

311. Resnick, H. (1978). It starts with people: Experiences in drug abuse prevention. Washington, DC: Porter, Novelli and Associates, Inc.

Examines and presents ways in which drug abuse prevention can be addressed in schools and communities. Strategies and educational techniques for prevention programs are emphasized, and organizational models for schools, communities, and minority groups are presented.

312. Riddle, M. (1982). Statement by Dr. M. Riddle, Coordinator, Substance Abuse Prevention, Fairfax County Public Schools before the U.S. Senate Committee on Labor and Human Resources. In: Hearing ... Ninety-Seventh Congress. Washington, DC: United States Government Printing Office.

Presents statistical data on the prevalence of alcohol and drug use by adolescents. Problems associated with this are discussed. Suggestions for prevention efforts are made.

313. Ritson, B. (1983). Treatment and evaluation of alcohol dependent children and adolescents. In: O. Jeanneret (Ed.), Alcohol and youth. Basel, Switzerland: S. Karger.

Discusses the risk factors associated with the development of alcohol problems among young people. The alcohol dependence syndrome is delineated. Recommendations for prevention through coordination of agency efforts are made.

314. Robins, L. (1973). The Vietnam drug user returns: Final report. Washington, DC: Special Action Office for Drug Abuse Prevention.

Presents the results of an evaluation of returning veterans from the Vietnam conflict. The evaluation covers many variables including a comparison of pre- and post-Vietnam variables. The report concludes with recommendations by study subjects that indicates what they feel the armed services can and should do to lessen drug-related activities.

315. Roessler, R., and others. (1976). Drug dependence and its treatment. Washington, DC: American Psychological Association, Supplement Abstract Service.

Presents a composite of information on treatment and rehabilitation of drug abusers. The material is presented as an annotated bibliography with 123 references. A special focus is made on material published between the years 1970 to 1974.

316. Rokeach, M. (1983). Value approach to the prevention and reduction of drug abuse. In: Preventing adolescent drug abuse: Intervention strategies. Rockville, MD: National Institute on Drug Abuse.

Discusses theoretical considerations and research on the values approach to prevention education. This method combines its efforts by providing both primary and secondary prevention strategies simultaneously.

317. Rosenblatt, J. (1982). Teenage drinking. In: H. Grimlin (Ed.), Youth problems. Washington, DC: Congressional Quarterly.

Presents an editorial research report on teenage drinking and discusses various topics related to this.

318. Ryan, W. (1974). A school-based drug abuse prevention program: An evaluation. Journal of drug education, 4(1), 61-66.

Presents the findings of an evaluation that measured the effect on self-regard of students' and teachers' perceptions of self-regard for these same students. Results indicate that there was an increase in cohesiveness and a subsequent increase in self-regard.

319. Ryser, P. (1983). Students and drug abuse. Journal of school health, 53(7), 435-436.

Presents emergency room contact information which indicates an increase in contacts for drug and alcohol related incidents. The author concludes that school health professionals and counselors must be alerted to student drug overdoses to assist students confronted with the idea of suicide.

320. Saltman, J. (1983). Teenagers and alcohol: Patterns and dangers. New York, NY: Public Affairs Committee.

Discusses the nature of teenage drinking, drinking and driving, why teenagers drink, as well as treatment and prevention issues related to teenagers.

* Samuels, D., and Samuels, M. (1975). The complete handbook of peer counseling. An authorative guide for the organization, training, implementation and evaluation of a peer counseling program. Miami, FL: Fiesta Publishing.

See No. 131.

321. Santa Cruz County Superintendent of Schools, California. (1973). Educational simulations: A project report, new approaches for behaviorally exceptional youth. Santa Cruz, CA: Author.

Describes the effectiveness of simulation games on the students of 19 corrective schools in Santa Cruz, California. The evaluation resulted in positive conclusions regarding the usefulness of the games and specific recommendations as to the most appropriate simulations by type of student and student grade level.

322. Schaeffer, G., and others. (1982). The effects of three years of participation in a primary prevention program on elementary school students. Napa, CA: Pacific Institute for Research and Evaluation.

Presents an evaluation of a primary prevention program that consisted of two years of the Magic Circle on the Human Development Program and one year of Jigsaw, a structured peer teaching model. The program was designed to influence students' social and emotional development as well as to enable them to take a more active role in the teaching/learning process. No significant findings were reported, in fact the program appeared to have a negative effect on the female student participants.

323. Schaps, E., and others. (1980). A process and outcome evaluation of an affective teacher training primary prevention program. Napa, CA: Pacific Institute for Research and Evaluation.

Describes a comprehensive teacher training model that was designed to teach effective classroom management through various communication, problem solving, and self-esteem enhancement techniques. Process evaluation data are presented.

324. Schlegal, A. (1981, April). National Committee for Protection Against Alcoholism. Paper presented at the European Youth Center Study Session, Strasbourg, France.

Presents a report of an International Good Templar Youth Federation Seminar. In addition, the extent of the alcoholism problem in France is described. Alcohol education projects are outlined.

325. Schluetter, W. (1980). Alcohol, drugs or alternatives: A film discussion guide. Minneapolis, MN: University of Minnesota, Continuing Education in Social Work.

Provides a follow-up and discussion guide for the concepts presented in the film, "Alcohol, drugs or alternatives." Includes background information on adolescent alcohol and drug misuse, a description of the film, and a series of discussion topics related to the film.

326. Schuchard, M. (1982). National parents' movement for drug free youth. In: PRIDE Southeast Drug Conference Proceedings, 1980 and 1981. Atlanta, GA: PRIDE.

Discusses how the drug and alcohol abuse epidemic among youth in the United States is perceived by and affects other countries. The role and responsibility of parents, schools, and communities in recognizing and addressing this problem are described.

327. Schuchard, M. (1983, September). Educating for prevention. In: Proceedings of the Fourth World Congress for the Prevention of Alcoholism and Drug Dependency. Nairobi, Kenya.

Asserts that the most pressing world health issue at present demands an appeal to mothers and fathers concerning alcohol and drug abuse among their children. The author suggests that parents form a parents-peer network, form guidelines for their children concerning social activities, and develop recreation programs as a means of prevention.

328. Seabright, C. (1973). A look at some current programs. Journal of drug education, 3(2), 127-140.

Describes some drug prevention programs in terms of philosophy, orientation, comprehensiveness, and audience. Conclusions include recommendations, opinions, and suggestions for development of a model prevention program.

329. Segal, B. (1983). Drugs and youth: A review of the problem. International journal of the addictions, 18(3), 429-433.

Presents research concerning the motives adolescents have for using drugs and alcohol. Discusses the implications of these findings for primary and secondary prevention efforts.

330. Seidenschnur, P. (1981). Young people's prevention and interventon manual. Little Rock, AR: Arkansas Highway Safety Program.

Provides knowledge and skills for young adults, which they should be able to employ in their daily life and interactions with others. Discusses the maladaptive functions of alcohol and drug abuse.

331. Sexter, J., Sullivan, A., Wepner, S., and Denmark, R. (1984). Substance abuse: Assessment of the outcomes of activities and activity clusters in school-based prevention. International journal of the addictions, 19(1), 79-92.

Examines the relationship between prevention activities in schools and drug abusing behaviors of students. The review included data from programs that represented different approaches to prevention. One-to-one staff student sessions and the availability of other students to provide direct help for students were activities reported as being associated with less abuse.

332. Shute, R. (1975). The impact of peer pressure on the verbally expressed drug attitudes of male college students. Paper presented at the Annual Meeting of the American Educational Research Association, Washington, DC.

Describes the role of peer pressure and group norms as they relate to the drug-using behaviors of the college students studied. Findings indicate that these students were most likely to adhere to the group norms as they related to drug using behavior.

333. Sieber, J., and others. (1976). The effects of learning when to be uncertain on children's knowledge and use of drug. R and D memorandum No. 144. Stanford, CA: Stanford University, Center for Research and Development in Teaching.

Presents the findings of an investigation into the long term effects of school-based drug abuse prevention curriculum. The authors present the research methodology, procedures, and the curriculum offered. Findings revealed that drug abuse prevention curriculum assisted students in differentiating between uncertainty about drugs, both hard and soft. Another valuable outcome is the effect of training on subsequent drug choice. Further findings indicated that significant change was noted from relatively short classroom training that did not contain information directly about drugs. Authors suggest strategies for future development of prevention efforts.

334. Simpson, D., and Santos De Barona, M. (1983). Drug abuse prevention for high risk youth in Texas. Texas Department of Community Affairs bulletin, 10(3), 4-7.

Describes the prevention efforts funded by the Texas Department of Community Affairs. Presents demographic data relative to clients receiving services, the problems that these clients have reported and other information reflecting the high risk environment of this population.

335. Smith, B. (1973). Values clarification in drug education: A comparative study. Journal of drug education, 3(4), 369-376.

Compares the effectiveness of two methods of teaching drug education to pre-service elementary school teachers. The two methods were the traditional teacher-confined approach and the values clarification group-centered approach. Findings indicate that the values clarification approach was superior in all ways measured.

* Smith, C. (1971). Drug education: Reasons and failures. Journal of drug education, 1(4), 373-389.

See No. 521.

336. Smith, E. (1981). Adolescent drug abuse and alcoholism: Directions for the school and the family. Urban education, 16(3), 311-322.

Examines the nature and extent of adolescent drug abuse and alcoholism. Discusses the etiology of adolescent drug abuse and drinking patterns. The social and psychological factors that lead to various drug addictive behaviors are explored. The author presents various treatment approaches that have been used with young people. Special attention is placed on drug abusing family systems, and the roles of the school and the community in preventing drug abuse.

* Social Advocates for Youth. (1978). Early age prevention of alcohol abuse project: Final report. San Francisco, CA: Author.

See No. 134.

* Solis, J. and Johnson, C. (1983). Comprehensive community programs for drug abuse implications of the Community Heart Disease Prevention Programs for future research. In: Preventing adolescent drug abuse: Intervention strategies. Rockville, MD: National Institute on Drug Abuse.

See No. 513.

337. Soroka, J. (1973). Coping with Newark's drug abuse dilemma. Journal of school health, 43(2), 126-128.

Describes the efforts to develop a drug prevention program in the Newark, New Jersey school system. Presents suggestions for improvement for more effective services.

338. Spivak, H. (1978). Health problems in the elementary school. National elementary principal, 57(2), 19-22.

Discusses several health issues that include, among others, drug and alcohol prevention efforts. The author contends that prevention efforts must begin in elementary schools.

339. Stainback, R., and Rogers, R. (1983). Identifying effective components of alcohol abuse prevention programs: Effects of fear appeals, message style, and source expertise. International journal of the addictions, 18(3), 393-405.

Findings indicate that there was positive results from the fear campaign. Implications are discussed for implementing these principles and for designing investigations of alcohol abuse prevention programs.

340. Stepien, H. (1979). Preventive action among children and adolescents. Problemy Alkoholizmu, 26(3), 4-8.

Describes prevention activities that include summer camps and other extracurricular activities. The author suggests that alcohol misuse is rooted in morally and materially backward families and that the solution to prevention is to change the attitude toward alcohol use among adults.

341. Strategy Council on Drug Abuse, Washington DC. (1974). Federal strategy for drug abuse and drug traffic prevention. Washington, DC: U.S. Government Printing Office.

Describes the initiatives developed by the government for prevention efforts. The project is built upon prevention services, criminal justice efforts, and international cooperation.

342. Striet, F., and Nicolich, M. (1977). Myths versus data on American Indian drug abuse. Journal of drug education, 7(2), 117-122.

Presents the findings from a drug and alcohol use prevalence study conducted on, and by, Montana Indians. Findings indicate that culture transmission may be helpful as a means of prevention. Recommendations for future research and for prevention needs are made.

343. Swanson, J. (1974). Junior high student evaluations of drug education by values and tradition oriented teachers. Journal of drug education, 4, 43-50.

Reports the results of student impressions of teachers trained in two different teaching styles: traditional and values clarification. The results were mixed, and it is concluded that a mix of the two approaches is best.

344. Swanson, J. (1978). The "No Win": Drug education evaluation problems. Journal of drug education, 8(2), 125-129.

Discusses the difficulty of prevention efforts in achieving their stated goals due to the confusion on the goals of prevention and treatment. The authors note that drug abuse prevention is in the domain of education and give new models for evaluating such goals.

* Swisher, J., and others. (1973). Four approaches to drug abuse prevention among college students. Journal of college student personnel, 13(3), 231-235.

See No. 139.

345. Swisher, J., and others. (1972). Experimental comparison of four approaches to drug abuse prevention among ninth and eleventh graders. Journal of counseling psychology, 19(4), 328-332.

Presents findings from a study that evaluated the effect of various prevention approaches on the behaviors of students from grades nine and eleven and compares these various approaches. Findings indicate that knowledge about drugs can be transmitted as effectively to students through traditional classroom techniques, through relationship group counseling or model reinforcement group counseling.

346. Swisher, J., and Horman, R. (1968). Evaluation of Temple University's drug abuse prevention program. Philadelphia, PA: Temple University.

Evaluates a university-wide drug abuse prevention program that included undergraduates, graduates, and staff. The program evaluation included pre- and post-testing. The report describes this prevention effort as a success and attributes the development of the Drug Education Activities Project to provide drug education, referral, and research services. Examples of pre- and post-tests, and data tables.

347. Swisher, J., and Horman, R. (1970). Drug abuse prevention. Journal of college student personnel, 2(5), 337-340.

Presents the results of the impact of Temple University's program entitled A Retreat on the Hazards of Drug Abuse. The authors refer to the program as effective but offer no empirical data.

348. Swisher, J., and Warner, R. (1971). A study of four approaches to drug abuse prevention. Final report. Washington, DC: Department of Health, Education and Welfare.

Compares the effectiveness of four approaches to drug abuse prevention. These are health education classes dealing with drug abuse, group counseling using model reinforcement, and a role model who has not abused drugs in addition to health education classes, and group counseling using model reinforcement with a role model who is a recovering addict. None of the models proved significantly different.

349. Swiss Institute for Alcoholism Prevention. (1982). Newsletter. October 29, 1982. Lausanne, Switzerland: Author.

Presents articles on the following topics: the role of parents in restricting alcohol use by children and adolescents; findings from a survey on alcohol habits amongst the Swiss; permissible blood levels; comparative statistics on alcoholic beverage consumption in Switzerland.

* Texas Education Agency. (1973). A framework for crime prevention and drug education in

Texas: Desirable student outcomes. Austin, TX: Author.

See No. 486.

350. Thomas, D. (1979). Problem of drinking. Nome, AK: Norton Sound Health Corporation.

Presents a workbook written for delegates from three Bering Straits villages who asked for workshops on alcohol problems. Contains information on alcohol and drinking problems, and exercises to be completed by parents, students, and other villagers.

* Thompson, E., Smith-Dijulio, K. and Matthews, T. (1982). Social control theory: Evaluating a model for the study of adolescent alcohol and drug use. Youth and society, 13(3), 303-32.

See No. 411.

351. Thomson, M. (1981). Austin's Drug-Alcohol Diversion Program. Police Chief, 48, 48-49.

Discusses alcoholism as a disease and describes an education prevention program that uses the disease concept of addiction, offered in Austin, Minnesota.

352. Toborg, M., Levin, D., Milkman, R., and Center, L. (1976). Treatment Alternatives to Street Crime (TASC) Projects, National evaluation programs, Phase I: Summary report. Washington, DC: National Institute of Law Enforcement and Criminal Justice.

Describes the TASC Projects that have as their goal the diversion of adolescent drug abusers that have come into contact with the criminal justice system. Project staff interview clients and refer these clients to appropriate treatment programs within their area and offer subsequent follow-up to ensure that clients are in compliance with program guidelines and criteria. The authors note that the lack of follow-up data of the treatment outcomes for TASC clients hampered the evaluation outcome.

353. Toohey, J., Valenzuela, G., and Dezelsky, T. (1981). Evaluating the feasibility of Spanish language drug and substance education program. Journal of drug education, 11(2), 179-184.

Presents the findings of an evaluation that measured the success and effects of a prevention program developed for Hispanic agencies. Findings concluded that Spanish-speaking agencies could use the student guide and the instructor's manual as a tool for drug education with their own staff conducting the program.

* Torrence, W., and Hanna, M. (1981). Administrative planning for a fusion of systems: Where prevention and treatment must merge. In: A.J. Schecter (Ed.), Drug dependence and alcoholism. Volume 2: Social behavior issues. New York, NY: Plenum Press.

See No. 489.

354. Trimble, J. Drug abuse prevention research needs among American Indians and Alaskan natives. White Cloud Journal, 3(3), 22-34.

Reviews the literature concerning prevalence and epidemiology of American Indian drug use and abuse and identifies the gaps in the research.

355. Utah Highway Safety Office. (1977). Juvenile court alcohol school evaluation interim report. Washington, DC: National Highway Traffic Safety Administration.

Describes the prevention efforts of the Utah Juvenile Court Alcohol School and compares this program with other prevention programs that are offered in the State of Utah. This is a preliminary report. The final report is noted to include recommendations to specialize the referral to treatment processes to lower recidivism rates.

356. Utley, E. (1982). Continued need for driver education. Journal of traffic safety education, 29(4), 9-25.

Discusses the implications of raising drinking ages to 21 as it relates to traffic accidents and drunk driving.

357. U.S. Department of Health and Human Services. (1980). Beyond the three R's: Training teachers for affective education. Rockville, MD: Author.

Presents ideas about the school's role and responsibility in the area of drug and alcohol prevention. Guidelines for training teachers to become more effective change agents are provided, including recommendations for schools of education, school systems, and teachers.

358. U.S. Department of Health and Human Services. (1981). The Door: A model youth center. Rockville, MD: Author.

Presents a program, The Door, which is a multifaceted youth center offering a broad range of services to youth in the city of New York, including, but not limited to, prevention services. Recommendations for developing and operating a service similar to The Door are provided.

359. U.S. Department of Transportation, National Highway Traffic Safety Administration. (1983). Alcohol and safety belt youth guide. Washington, DC: Author.

Discusses and presents a coordinated effort to be established to maintain the interest in combating drunk driving. Objectives, strategies, and activities are outlined for reducing drunk driving.

360. Valencia County Commission. (1974). Rio Grande Youth Care Center: Final report. Los Lunas, NM: Author.

Describes a counseling and referral center designed to reduce delinquency among the Chicanos in New Mexico. The evaluation indicated that the project has been successful in meeting its objectives.

361. Ventura, M., and Dundon, M. (1974). A challenging experience in canoeing and camping as a tool in approaching the drug problem. Journal of drug education, 4(1), 123-127.

Presents the findings of an evaluation on a prevention program modeled after the Outward Bound program. No significant findings are noted.

362. Vejnoska, J. (1982). Parent action groups: A prevention resource. Alcohol health and research world, 6(4), 13-17.

Discusses parents' attitudes to the use of alcohol and drugs by their children. Includes the development and activities of parent action groups as a prevention resource.

363. Vejnoska, J. (1982). Project Graduation seeks to reduce teen DWI incidents. Alcohol health and research world, 7(1), 33.

Describes the implementation of Project Graduation, a program developed to reduce drinking on graduation and prom nights. This project was developed by teachers, parents, students, and members of the business community in Montgomery County, Maryland.

364. Vejnoska, J. (1982). Putting the brakes on teenage drunk driving. Police chief, 49(12), 35-38.

Presents statistical data on drunk driving to describe the extent of the problem. Makes recommendations for the prevention of drunk driving.

365. Voas, R. (1974). Alcohol, drugs and young drivers. Washington, DC: National Highway Safety Administration.

Reviews the research literature on the relationship of drugs, alcohol, and driving among young people, university students, and a group of young criminals. The data shows that young people use drugs more than adults do, and that they drive under the influence of drugs and alcohol more readily than adults do.

366. Wallack, L. (1981). Winners: A primary prevention alcohol abuse program. Berkeley, CA: University of California School of Public Health, Research Group.

Describes a three-year effort in California to reduce alcohol consumption and alcohol-related problems. The program used mass media and community based education to achieve their stated goals.

367. Warner, R. (1973). Preventing drug abuse: Where are we now? Personnel and guidance journal, 51(8), 523-529.

Reviews research literature on prevention programs. Presents common themes which may prove helpful to counselors involved in the development and implementation of drug prevention programs.

368. Webb, R. (1974). Fear and communication. Journal of drug education, 4(1), 97-103.

Presents abstracts of important findings on the relationship between fear and communication. Attention is drawn to the conflicting nature of the evidence between the relationship to drug abuse and drug abuse prevention.

369. West, P., and others. (1976). Report on a needs assessment and evaluation of a drug education program. Van Nuys, CA: Los Angeles Valley College.

Describes the prevention program developed by the Los Angeles Valley College and evaluates the use of the services. The program described as a resource center with a training component. Suggestions for increasing use of such services are offered. Suggestions are made for other similar programs and how they can increase program use.

370. Wheeler, W. (1976). Blackness is my mental health: A mind set for black drug abuse prevention and treatment programs. Journal of non-white concerns in personnel and guidance, 4(2), 64-70.

Discusses the factors responsible for the failure of programs aimed at eliminating drug abuse in the black community. The author notes that this is due to the existing social and political systems and those blacks that support these. The author makes suggestions to deal with this problem.

371. White, J. (1983). American Indian youth alcohol and alcoholism prevention project. Dissertation abstracts international, 44(3), 878-A.

Describes the American Indian Center, established to alleviate some of the housing, education, medical, and unemployment problems of the American Indian population. As a prevention project, the center worked to reduce the stigma of alcoholism and to create a climate where young people would feel free to seek help. Results from a program evaluation indicate that knowledge can be increased and self-worth can be changed through the services offered through the center.

* Winger, J. (1979). Peer dynamic 1978-1979 evaluation report. Lincoln, NE: Nebraska State Department of Education.

See No. 414.

372. Wong, M. (1975, April). Different strokes: Models of drug abuse prevention. Paper presented at the Annual Meeting of the

American Educational Research Association, Washington, DC.

Describes models of drug abuse prevention programs deliniated in the literature over the prior six years, 1969 through 1975, and discusses the research related to these models.

373. Wunderlich, R., Lozes, J., and Lewis, J. (1974). Recidivism rates of group therapy participants and other adolescents processed by a juvenile court. Psychotherapy: Therapy, research, and practice, 11(3), 243-245.

Describes the evaluation of a short-term group therapy project for adolescent drug abusers and their parents. The goal of the project was to develop better communication skills so that families could be better able to handle future conflicts.

* Zucker, R., and Noll, R. (1982). Precursors and developmental influences on drinking and etiology from a longitudinal perspective. In: Alcohol and health monograph no. 1: Alcohol consumption and related problems. Washington, DC: Department of Health and Human Services.

See No. 415.

Peer Pressure

374. Appleby, A. (1981, March). Alternatives for adolescents. In: Proceedings of the First Pan-Pacific Conference on Drugs and Alcohol. Canberra, Australia.

Presents prevalence data on drug and alcohol usage among Australian youth. Briefly discusses reasons for such usage. Presents "realities" about drug abuse and adolescents as well as requisites to be considered for adolescents in treatment. Case reports are included to substantiate these considerations.

375. Beauvais, F., Oetting, E., and Edwards, R. (1982). Boredom, poor self-image, lead young Indian girl to drugs. NIHB health reporter, 3(2), 5-9.

Presents a case study of an 11-year-old Indian who chose to use drugs as a result of peer pressure and as a means of escaping problems. The authors generalize this experience to the larger Indian drug and alcohol problem and present material for prevention concerns.

376. Blount, W., and Dembo, R. (1984). Effect of perceived neighborhood setting on self-reported tobacco, alcohol, and marijuana use among inner city minority junior high school youth. International journal of the addictions, 19(2), 175-198.

Presents data gathered from a survey of youth from New York City's South Bronx neighborhoods. Findings indicate that there is a relationship between perception of neighborhood and drug usage; further, this seems to be a drug-specific relationship. Knowledge of friends' drug usage appeared to be highly predictive in drug use. The authors conclude that intervention and prevention efforts must not only be drug-specific but must proceed on many fronts simultaneously. Examples are presented.

377. Braucht, G. (1982). Problem drinking among adolescents: A review and analysis of psychosocial research. In: Alcohol and health monograph No. 4: Special population issues. Washington, DC: United States Government Printing Office.

Reviews research on the psychosocial correlates of adolescent problem drinking. Results of research are presented and discussed.

378. Brown, J., and Finn, P. (1982). Drinking to get drunk: Findings of a survey of junior and senior high school students. Journal of alcohol and drug education, 27(3), 13-25.

Findings indicate that the majority of youth that drank to get drunk denied that this was the effect of peer pressure and that they did it because of enjoyment. Implications of these behaviors and extreme alcohol consumption are discussed as they relate to educators, counselors, and parents.

* Cooper, C., and Walker, C. (1980). Peer dynamics Final Evaluation Report. 1979-1980, Part II. Lincoln, NE: Nebraska State Department of Education.

See No. 187.

379. Dawkins, M. (1981). Alcohol and drug survey among youth and adolescents in a descriptive summary. Washington, DC: Washington Area Council on Alcoholism and Drug Abuse, Inc.

Presents the findings of a city-wide survey to assess behavior and attitudes of youth in

Washington, DC, as they relate to alcohol. Findings indicate that the youth of the city follow many of the patterns of national figures. These figures are corroborated with figures of crime, health, and social service statistics.

380. Dembo, R., Schmeidler, J., Taylor, R., and Burgos, W. (1982). Supports for, and consequences of, early drug involvement among inner city junior high school youths living in three neighborhood settings. Journal of drug education, 12(3), 191-210.

Presents the findings of a survey to assess the prevalence of drug usage and reasons for such usage. The findings indicate that there is a relationship between perceived neighborhood setting and various supports for, and consequences of drug involvement. The authors indicate that the reasons youth use drugs should be the subject of future research to enhance and improve prevention programs.

381. Dorn, N. (1981). Youth culture in the U.K.: Independence and round drinking implications for health education. International journal of health education, 24(2), 77-82.

Discusses some of the reasons for youthful alcohol abuse. The authors indicate that the primary reason is peer pressure and the second is exposure to early and heavy drinking patterns from the media. Suggestions for consideration in changes in health education programs are made.

382. Dutton, D. (1982). Decisions, decisions, decisions. Albany, NY: Alcohol Education for Youth.

Provides information for student groups and group leaders, concerning the use of alcohol and drugs. The author presents resource materials to assist in the development of student sessions, including a reading list, pamphlets, and films.

383. Englander-Golden, P., and others. (1984, August). Say it straight: Adolescent substance abuse prevention training. Paper presented at the Annual Convention of the American Psychological Association, Toronto, Canada.

Describes the process and patterns of peer pressure and the role this has in drug abuse. It also includes an evaluation of the program Say It Straight, a prevention program for youth that is designed around and uses peer pressure in its efforts.

384. Forrest, G. (1983). How to cope with a teenage drinker: New alternatives and hope for parents and families. New York, NY: Atheneum.

Presents information for parents on the epidemic of teenage alcoholism. Major topics discussed are treatment alternatives, interpersonal skill building for family members, and the stages of recovery. Family roles that promote alcohol abuse and those that thwart alcohol abuse are delineated. The role of peer pressure in the development of the alcohol problem is discussed.

* General Research Corp. (1973). Evaluation of selected components of the Office of Education, "Help Communities Help Themselves," drug abuse prevention program. Washington, DC: United States Department of Health, Education, and Welfare.

See No. 98.

385. Harford, T. and Spiegler, D. (1982). Environmental influences in adolescent drinking. In: Alcohol and health monograph no. 4: Special populations issue. Washington, DC: United States Government Printing Office.

Discusses previously reported findings in adolescent drinking patterns and the roles of neighborhood and peer pressure. The authors make recommendations for future research.

386. Harford, T., Wechsler, H., and Rohman, M. (1983). Structural context of college drinking. Journal of studies on alcohol, 44(4), 722-732.

Presents the findings of a research project that studied the drinking settings and companions of college students. Suggestions are offered for further studies of the factors impacting the drinking behavior of college students.

* Haun, D. (1975). Where kids teach kids. Teacher, 92(7), 59-61.

See No. 9.

* Hedin, D., and Norem-Hebeisen, A. (1983). Influences on adolescent problem behavior: Causes, connections, and contexts. In: R. Isralowitz, and M. Singer (Eds.), Adolescent Substance Abuse: A guide to prevention and treatment. New York, NY: Haworth Press.

See No. 233.

387. Jaynes, J. and Rugg, C. (1983). Role of chemical abuse during adolescence. Focus on alcohol and drug abuse, 6(3), 16-17.

Discusses the role that alcohol plays in the overall development of adolescents. Also discussed is the difficulty of treating adolescents for alcohol problems. The authors note the role alcohol plays in the developmental process and the subsequent impediments in future stages of life. The authors conclude that treatment programs that plan on serving the adolescent population must be, philosophically, based on the view that adolescent chemical abuse is a "need meeting" process and must, therefore, facilitate ways that adolescents can meet these needs and developmental tasks in healthy, appropriate, and skill building ways.

* Koberl, I. (1981). Thoughts on drug prevention and prophylaxis. Wiener zeitschrift fuer such forschung, 4(1), 17-19.

See No. 260.

388. Krohn, M., Akers, R., Radosevich, M., and Lanza-Kaduce, L. (1982). Norm qualities and adolescent drinking and drug behavior: The effects of norm quality and reference group on using and abusing alcohol and marijuana. Journal of drug issues, 12(4), 343-359.

Presents the findings from a survey designed to investigate the effect of normative climate on use, patterns of use, and attitudes towards alcohol and marijuana among adolescents. Findings included that the most predictable variable is the norm quality of friends. Other variables included parents and religion.

* Lassey, M. and Carlson, J. (1981). Teenage drinking in Idaho's rural communities. Moscow, ID: University of Idaho College of Agriculture.

See No. 110.

389. Lee, E. (1983). Survey of knowledge, attitudes, and practices of fifth and eighth grade students regarding alcoholic beverages in urban parochial schools. Journal of alcohol and drug education, 28(2), 73-84.

Surveys the attitudes, knowledge, and practices of 3785 boys and girls in the fifth and eighth grades. Two grade levels were selected to identify increased influence in peer pressure and decreased influence in family value systems.

390. Libbey, P., and Blum, R. (1980). Adolescent voice on drinking and drugs: A developmental perspective. Minneapolis, MN: University of Minnesota, Adolescent Health Program.

Surveyed adolescents to examine moral

decision-making processes and feelings before, during, and after, first experiences with either drugs or alcohol. Personal experiences were placed within a four-stage developmental framework. The authors conclude that the core of the developmental crisis was a conflict between belonging and autonomy. These adolescents were found to shift their locus of decision-making from fear of parental punishment to a sense of shame in front of others.

391. McDonald, D. (1982). Progressive stages of teenage drug abuse. In: Pride Southeast Drug Conference Proceedings 1980 and 1981. Atlanta, GA: PRIDE.

Discusses the five stages of drug abuse observed in teenagers, and describes the role of parents and peers in enhancing and preventing drug abuse in teenagers.

392. Moberg, D., Robertson, J., Fischer, J., and Downs, W. (1982). Alcohol and other drug use by Dane County teenagers: Findings from a telephone survey. Madison, WI: University of Wisconsin.

Presents data from a survey of adolescents to assess the extent of alcohol and drug use among teenagers aged 13-17, the extent to which teenagers have had exposure to alcohol and drug abuse prevention, intervention, and treatment programs, to identify those willing to participate in a longitudinal study, and to test a variety of hypotheses concerning adolescent drug and alcohol use. Findings include the role that peer pressure has played in the development of drug and alcohol abuse problems.

* Morriss, R. (1983). Peer education teaches Minnesota teenagers the control factor in drinking and driving. Traffic Safety, 83(5), 6-8.

See No. 116.

393. Pascnke, W. (1970). The addictive cycle: A learning theory--peer group model. Corrective psychiatry and journal of social therapy, 16(1-4), 74-81.

Explores the psychological theories underlying the concepts of learning theory and peer group process. Inferences for utilization by prevention programs are made. Peer pressure is described as the most important aspect of early substance abuse. It may well be that peer pressure is the ingredient that can also prevent substance abuse.

* Plat, P. (1981). Alcohol in the school age child. Revue De L'Alcoolisme, 27(1), 31-42.

See No. 308.

394. Polzella, S., and Selinger, M. (1981). Teacher intervention for the adolescent substance abuser. Arlington, VA: Educational Document Reproduction Service.

Reviews adolescent development and considers the role of teachers in dealing with compulsive adolescent substance abusers. Suggestions for relationship building with the student are given.

395. PTA Today. (1982). How you can help your child make responsible decisions about drinking. PTA today, 7(4), 6-b.

Suggests ways parents can help their children make responsible decisions about drinking. Gives strategies for parents to assist their children in learning skill building skills. Indicates ways children and parents can deal with peer pressure.

396. Pulkkinen, L. (1982). Smoking and drinking among youth: A longitudinal study. Alkoholipolitiikka, 47(3), 139-146.

Presents the findings from a study of 135 subjects studied at the ages of eight, fourteen, and twenty. Findings indicate that there are age-related predicators that help identify potential smokers and drinkers. The author concludes that the findings are highly significant towards peer pressure being a primary causative factor leading to substance abuse.

397. Rachal, J., Maisto, S., Guess, L., and Hubbard, R. (1982). Alcohol use among youth. In: Alcohol and health monograph No. 1: Alcohol consumption and related problems. Washington, DC: United States Department of Health and Human Services.

Addresses questions concerning the extent and nature of adolescent drinking behaviors. Findings include demographic information, social and behavioral correlates, and descriptive results over the last 25 years, as well as specifying future research needs. The authors conclude that adolescent alcohol use is a developmental phenomenon which teenagers must address.

398. Recchia, C. (1982, April 4). Treating youthful alcoholics. News-American, Baltimore, MD.

Describes Baltimore's Youth Alcohol Program. This program is directed at children and teenagers. They have identified target populations as teenagers, pregnant women, and adult women.

* Regional Health Planning Council of the North Central Texas Council of Governments. (1975). Proposed 1975 North Central Texas regional plan for the prevention and treatment of alcohol abuse and alcoholism: A summary. Arlington, TX: Author.

See No. 127.

399. Rehrer, R. (1982). Now what do I do? A guide on alcohol and drugs for youth. St. Louis, MO: Concordia Publishing House.

Presents material that can be used as a guide for youth and as a resource for parents. The author describes the effects of peer pressure and other influences that are exerted on young people to initiate drug use. Provides a list of materials on drugs and alcohol for parents and teachers.

400. Rooney, J. (1983). Influence of informal control sources upon adolescent alcohol use and problems. American journal of drug and alcohol abuse, 9(2), 233-245.

Presents the results of a survey to study and identify the sources that exert formal control on adolescent alcohol use. The findings indicate that the greatest control factor is peer pressure.

401. Rozelle, G., and Gonzalez, G. (1979). A peer-facilitated course on alcohol abuse: An innovative approach to prevention on the college campus. Journal of alcohol and drug education, 25(1), 20-30.

Examines curriculum approaches to determine effectiveness in increasing college students' responsibility toward alcohol. An experiential peer-facilitated approach decreased negative consequences of drinking. Shows that an academic course on alcohol abuse can be an important part of a campus alcohol abuse prevention program.

* Ryan, W. (1976). Project youth: An approach to drug abuse. Guidance and counseling, 10(4), 270-278.

See No. 19.

402. Saltman, J. (1983). Teenagers and alcohol: Patterns and dangers. New York, NY: Public Affairs Committee.

Discusses teenage alcohol use and includes the following topics: nature of adolescent alcohol use; drinking and driving; why teenagers drink; control of drinking and driving; and treatment and prevention.

* Samuels, D., and Samuels, M. (1975). The complete handbook of peer counseling. An authorative guide for the organization, training, implementation and evaluation of a peer counseling program. Miami, FL: Fiesta Publishing Corp.

See No. 131.

* Schuchard, M. (1982). National parents' movement for drug-free youth. In: PRIDE Southeast Drug Conference Proceedings, 1980 and 1981. Atlanta, GA: PRIDE.

See No. 326.

403. Scoles, P. and Fine, E. (1981). Substance abuse patterns among youthful drinking drivers. Alcoholism clinical experience, 5, 167.

Describes the need for prevention efforts that include complications of polydrug abuse, peer pressure, and primary prevention.

404. Shada, M., and Winger, J. (1978). Peer dynamics: 1977-78 Evaluation report. Lincoln, NE: Nebraska State Department of Education.

Presents the findings of the evaluation of the second year of services offered to reduce the incidence of destructive risk taking behavior amongst school age youth. Data indicates a decrease in number of contacts with police and a notable drop in discipline referrals amongst students. Recommendations for program improvements are included.

405. Shore, R. (1983). Social ease in drinking situations among college students. International journal of the addictions, 18(6), 875-880.

Discusses an investigation on two midwestern college campuses where situations involving drinking and various student characteristics were studied. Findings indicate that early experiences with alcohol may influence student ease in drinking situations and that present exposure to drinking situations is also suggested as a factor in student ease.

406. Shore, E., Rivers, P., and Berman, J. (1983). Resistance by college students to peer pressure to drink. Journal of studies on alcohol, 44(2), 352-361.

Presents the results of a study designed to investigate college students' resistance to drink and their desire to refrain from drinking. The authors conclude that programs aimed at the modification of drinking behavior among college students might benefit from consideration of the environment of the specific college.

* Shute, R. (1975). The impact of peer pressure on the verbally expressed drug attitudes of male college students. Paper presented at the Annual Meeting of the American Educational Research Association, Washington, DC, 1975.

See No. 332.

407. Spazzapan, B., and DeVanna, M. (1981). Cultural aspects of alcoholic habits in lower middle schools. Minerva psichiatrica, 22(4), 177-182.

Reports on a study of 879 students, aged 11-15, in Gorizia, Italy. It is concluded that adolescent drinking is most impacted by parental teaching and peer influence.

408. Stumphauzer, J. (1983). Learning not to drink: Adolescents and abstinence. Journal of drug education, 13(1), 39-48.

Discusses a survey of nondrinking adolescents. Findings indicate that adolescents who did not drink were those that were influenced towards this decision by parents and peers who did not drink. Self-reinforcement appeared to play a role in this behavior in the form of feeling proud. The author discusses the issue of using nondrinking and nondrug using adolescents as teachers in drug education and prevention programs.

409. Stumphauzer, J., and Perez, P. (1982). Learning to drink. II. Peer survey of normal adolescents. International journal of the addictions, 17(8), 1363-1372.

Presents the findings of a study where 100 adolescents who reported drinking regularly were surveyed by their peers. Results support the notion that adolescent alcohol use is reinforced by both drug effect and peer approval. Implications for further research are given. Issues of treatment and prevention are discussed.

410. Svobodny, L. (1982). Biographical, self-concept, and educational factors among chemically dependent adolescents. Adolescence, 17(68), 847-853.

Presents the findings of a study where adolescents who entered a residential chemical dependency treatment program were studied as to the precursors of their drug abuse. A control group of randomly chosen adolescents from the local high school were selected. Findings indicate that poor family interaction, peer influence to use drugs, low self-esteem, inadequacy in relating to others, and an inability to cope with problems were factors that influenced their drug abuse.

411. Thompson, E., Smith-Dijulio, K., and Matthews, T. (1982). Social control theory: Evaluating a model for the study of adolescent alcohol and drug use. Youth and society, 13(3), 303-326.

Discusses the findings of a study designed to explore the utility of social control theory for explaining adolescent drug and alcohol use. The most significant indication of substance abuse was found to be peer influence, while social control theory variables were most useful in discriminating illicit drug and polydrug use. Treatment implications of these findings are reviewed.

412. Torres, D. (1982). Youth and alcohol abuse: A continuing phenomenon. Journal of alcohol and drug education, 27(2), 74-82.

Discusses youth and their relationship with alcohol. It is suggested that teenagers consume alcohol for a variety of reasons. The author states that it is this alcohol usage that can lead to alcohol dependence and can cause interference in normal relationships with others.

413. Wenk, E. (1973). Peer conducted research: A novel approach in drug education. Paper presented at the First International Congress on Drug Education, Montreux, Vd., Switzerland.

High school students researched specific topics amongst their peers. Findings from the students' study are listed and possibilities for further use of the model are examined.

414. Winger, J. (1979). Peer dynamics 1978-79 evaluation report. Lincoln, NE: Nebraska State Department of Education.

Presents the findings of the first year evaluation of a program to reduce the incidence of destructive risk-taking behaviors. Background research indicates that the single most important indicator of drug abuse is the role that peer pressure plays in the final choice to use drugs.

* Wong, M. (1975, April). Different strokes: Models of drug abuse prevention. Paper presented at the Annual Meeting of the American Educational Research Association, Washington, DC.

See No. 372.

415. Zucker, R., and Noll, R. (1982). Precursors and developmental influences on drinking and etiology from a longitudinal perspective. In: Alcohol and health monograph No. 1: Alcohol consumption and related problems. Washington, DC: Department of Health and Human Services.

Discusses a model for research that had as its objective etiological influences of drug and alcohol problems. Findings indicate that four classes of influences were revealed: sociocultural and community influences; primary group influences (family); secondary group influences (peer group); and intraindividual influences. The author suggests that future research use these four variables as a basis.

CURRICULA/MATERIALS

* Addiction Research Foundation. (1979). Core Knowledge in the Drug Field. Ontario, Canada: Author.

See No. 79.

416. Adix, R., Kelly, T., and Rosenthal, D. (1984). Substance abuse prevention: A developmental skills approach. Journal for specialists in group work, 9(1), 32-37.

Describes a school-based prevention program that uses group work and developmental skill building as a prevention process. The program is curriculum bound and focused towards an elementary school population. It has components for teaching staff as well as parents. Curriculum experiences are decision making, identification of alternatives for substance abuse, information about substance abuse, interpersonal skills building, and stress management.

417. Allen, L., and others. (1976). Health education for special children: Primary EMR. Albany, NY: New York State Education Department.

Developed for teachers and school administrators in special education, the guide offers information on planning a health education program for educable mentally handicapped children at the primary level. Among many other topics are drug and alcohol prevention projects. The authors have also developed similar curricula for other levels of exceptional students.

* American Association for Health, Physical Education, and Recreation. (1969). Research book for drug abuse information. Washington, DC: National Science Teachers Association.

See No. 287.

* Anderson, D.S., and Gadaleto, A.F. (1976). That happy feeling--An innovative model for a campus alcohol education program. Ratford, VA: Ratford University.

See No. 1.

418. Babst, D., Miran, M., and Koval, M. (1976). The relationship between friends' marijuana use, family cohesion, school interest and drug abuse prevention. Journal of drug education, 6(1), 23-41.

Examines the differences in responses of rural and suburban high school students to various drug abuse prevention strategies, so that some sensitivity to differences in audience's needs can be known for planning. Results showed that students most involved with drugs were those least receptive to traditional educational programs. Results also indicated that except for the rates of drug abuse, rural and suburban student responses were similar. It concludes that peer, family and school factors may be better predictors than rural and suburban distinctions.

419. Baltimore City Public Schools. (1969). Drug Abuse Education, Grades 5, 7, 9. Baltimore, MD: Author.

Presents the curriculum guide developed for the three mentioned grades. Each unit outlines the curriculum content and learning activities for each of the three grades.

420. Beauvais, F. (1980). Preventing drug abuse among American Indian young people. Ft. Collins, CO: Colorado State University.

Presents a summary report of existing research on drug abuse in American Indian communities. The author suggests ways to combat this problem and further describes different kinds of drugs and their effects.

421. Bedworth, D. (1973). Health education: A humanizing catalyst for drug abuse prevention. Illinois teacher for contemporary roles, 16(3), 195-198.

Describes the teacher's role in prevention of substance abuse through health education programs.

422. Bensley, M. (1974). Coronado Plan: Teacher's guide. San Diego, CA: Pennant.

Describes four teachers guides which attempt to fuse drug abuse instruction with a valuing program based on the Lowell-Rucker categories. The approach describes attempts to inculcate specific values in students.

423. Berberian, R., Gross, C., Lovejoy, J., and Paparella, S. (1976). The effectiveness of drug education programs: A critical review. Health education monographs, 4(4), 377-398.

Reviews published studies of drug abuse prevention programs. Notes that most of the studies did not evaluate actual drug using behaviors. Those claiming reliable results are noted to be contradictory in their conclusions. It is suggested that school-based programs, henceforward, be designed and conducted as experiments with controlled manipulation of relevant variables.

424. Brodie, P., and others. (1976). Health education for special children: Intermediate ED-LD. Albany, NY: New York State Education Department.

Presents a curriculum guide offering information on developing health education programs for emotionally disturbed or learning disabled children in intermediate grades. Among other topics, the issue of substance abuse prevention is presented.

425. Brodie, P., and others. (1976). <u>Health education for special children: Intermediate EMR</u>. Albany, NY: New York State Education Department.

Presents a curriculum guide offering information on developing health education programs for educable mentally handicapped children in intermediate grades. Among other topics, the issue of substance abuse prevention is presented.

426. Brodie, P., and others. (1976). <u>Health education for special children: Junior High EMR</u>. Albany, NY: New York State Education Department.

Presents a curriculum guide offering information on developing health education programs for educable mentally handicapped children in junior high school. Among other topics, the issue of substance abuse prevention is presented.

427. Brodie, P., and others. (1976). <u>Health education for special children: Intermediate TMP</u>. Albany, NY: New York State Education Department.

Presents a curriculum guide offering information on developing health education programs for special education children in intermediate grades. Among other topics, the issue of substance abuse prevention is presented.

428. Brundage, E., and others. (1976). <u>Health education for special children: Secondary ED-LD</u>. Albany, NY: New York State Education Department.

Presents a curriculum guide offering information on developing health education programs for emotionally disturbed or learning disabled students in the secondary grades. Among other topics, the issue of substance abuse prevention is presented.

429. Brundage, E., and others. (1976). Health education for special children: Secondary TMR. Albany, NY: New York State Education Department.

Describes a curriculum guide offering information on developing health education programs for special education students in the secondary grades. Among other topics, the issue of substance abuse prevention is presented.

430. Brundage, E., and others. (1976). Health education for special children: Senior High EMR. Albany, NY: New York State Education Department.

Describes a curriculum guide offering information on developing health education programs for educable mentally handicapped students in senior high school. Among other topics, the issue of substance abuse prevention is presented.

431. Carlisle Area School District. (1970). A Program for the prevention of drug abuse, Kindergarten-Adult. Carlisle, PA: Author.

Identifies the school's responsibility and program with regard to drug education and the prevention of drug abuse among young people. Provides general overviews that schools may take and suggest pupil-teacher activities for reinforcement of suggested goals and objectives in curriculum materials for K-3 and 4-6 grades.

* Center of Alcohol Studies. (1980). Recent topics in alcohol studies. New Brunswick, NJ: Rutgers University.

See No. 589.

* Center for Disease Control. (1976). The Bureau of Health Education's Elementary

School Health Curriculum Project, Berkeley Model, and the American Lung Association--Bureau of Health Education's Primary Grades Health Curriculum Project, Seattle Model. Atlanta, GA: Author.

See No. 177.

* The Center for Youth Development and Research. (1980). The youth work bibliography. St. Paul, MN: Author.

See No. 590.

432. Clements, M. (1978). Health and drug education--A regional approach. Educational leadership, 35(4), 314-317.

Describes the Values Clarification Project and the Berkeley Health Curriculum Project, two educational programs being used by southwest Iowa schools in order to reduce drug abuse.

* Coleman, J. (1978). Deviant subcultures and the schools. In: Theoretical perspectives on school crime. Vol. I. Washington, DC: Department of Health, Education and Welfare.

See No. 501.

* Cook, R., Lawrence, H., Morse, C., and Roehl, J. (1984). An evaluation of the alternatives approach to drug abuse prevention. International journal of the addictions, 19(7), 767-787.

See No. 184.

433. Cooperative Educational Service Agency 8. (1977). Teacher activity package: Drug information. Grades 2-6. Appleton, WI: Author.

Contains factual materials for the teacher to use with primary and intermediate students. It is designed for use in conjunction with having students learn more about themselves, their values, and decision-making. The materials are geared towards several essential areas of drug prevention education, helping the child know what constitutes a drug and how drug abuse is defined, classifying household medicines, and understanding the different effects of major drugs. The overall design of the activities is to promote the proper use of drugs by the students and to help them consider for themselves the propriety of using or abusing drugs.

* Creighton, H. (1975). Health education encounters. New York, NY: J. Wiley & Sons.

See No. 520.

* Cuenot, R. (1982). Evaluation of effectiveness of a one-time alcohol abuse prevention education assembly. Psychological reports, 51(2), 440-442.

See No. 190.

434\. Dembo, R., et al. (1978). Neighborhood relationships and drug involvement among inner-city junior high school youths: Implications for drug education and prevention programming. Journal of drug education, 8(3), 231-252.

Presents the findings of a survey taken amongst inner-city youth in high school. It assessed the relationship between students' attitudes towards their neighborhood, leisure time activities, and self-esteem with substance abuse. Findings imply that substance abuse prevention programs will be enhanced by a focus on life-style commitment, rather than on such things as drug use, per se.

435\. Denton, C. (1972). Youngsters get a marionette message. Pennsylvania education, 3(4), 19-22.

Describes a program that uses marionettes to

develop a sense of morality in decision making. The author notes that if children can be taught to better define right and wrong within their own value system, they will be better able to make decisions on major problems such as drug and alcohol use.

436. Devens, D. (1977). Continuing education in chemical dependency focuses on adult learners. Journal of drug education, 7(2), 141-148.

Describes a program that trains allied health professionals in chemical dependency. The program is based on the concept that adult learners are responsible to plan, develop, implement, and evaluate their own learning experiences.

437. Dippo, J., (Ed.). (1975). Steps toward healthy growth. Health education curriculum guide; Grades K-3. Homer, NY: Cortland-Madison Board of Cooperative Educational Services.

Covers all areas of health education including chemical abuse and use. Each chapter is broken into specific areas and contains an overview of the material, list of instructional objectives, major concepts, content outline, list of learning and evaluation activities.

438. Dippo, J., (Ed.). (1975). Steps toward healthy growth. Health education curriculum guide; Grades 4-6. Homer, NY: Cortland-Madison Board of Cooperative Educational Services.

Presents materials, learning objectives, and all other related materials for the instruction of a health education program for grades 4-6. The author uses the same format as in the other curriculum guides that she has developed for other grade levels.

439. Dippo, J., (Ed.). (1975). Steps toward healthy growth. Health education curriculum

guide; Grades 7-9. Homer, NY: Cortland-Madison Board of Cooperative Educational Services.

Presents materials, learning objectives, and all other related materials for the instruction of a health education program for grades 7-9. The author uses the same format as in the other curriculum guides that she has developed for other grade levels.

440. Dippo, J. (Ed.). (1975). Steps toward healthy growth. Health education curriculum guide; Grades 10-12. Homer, NY: Cortland-Madison Board of Cooperative Educational Services.

Presents materials, learning objectives, and all other related materials for the instruction of a health education program for grades 10-12. The author uses the same format as in the other curriculum guides that she has developed for other grade levels.

* Dorn, N. (1981). Youth culture in the U.K.: Independence and round drinking implications for health education. International journal of health education, 24(2), 77-82.

See No. 381.

* Dutton, D. (1982). Decisions, decisions, decisions. Albany, NY: Alcohol Education for Youth.

See No. 382.

441. Education Developmental Center, Inc. (1982). Protecting oneself and others: Smoking, drinking, and drugs. Newton, MA: Author.

Presents a module for prevention education from a health education curriculum, TMTH Program. The goal of the program is to provide secondary school students with knowledge, skills, and an understanding that will enable them to act on behalf of themselves and others in a health enhancing way.

442. Edwards, G., and Holloway, J. (1975). Drug education: A misnomer. Journal of research and development in education, 8(2), 83-95.

Argues that prevention programs must include a focus on the psychosocial causes of drug abuse in addition to the educational issues. Several program components are discussed. These being individual and group counseling, group rap sessions, workshops for different target groups, peer leadership, big brother/ sister, hotline services, and curriculum development. A multidisciplinary team approach is presented for the staff pattern of such a program.

443. Eiseman, S. (1971). Education about narcotics and dangerous drugs: A challenge to our schools. Journal of drug education, 1(2), 177-185.

Describes the role of the school as a preventive agent of drug abuse. It is suggested that abuse may be curtailed by developing a comprehensive plan utilizing thought, inquiry, analysis, evaluation, and decision-making. A method is presented for using multiple disciplines to reinforce the drug education program, thus building up a thrust within the existing curriculum.

444. Finn, P., and Platt, J. (1987). Alcohol and alcohol safety, Volume II of II. A curriculum manual for elementary level. A teacher's activities guide. Rockville, MD: National Institute on Alcohol Abuse and Alcoholism.

Describes curricula and activites for teachers in elementary schools for the prevention of substance abuse. The guide is well organized and includes individual, group, and self-contained instructional methods.

445. Franklin, J. (1985). Alternative education as substance abuse prevention. Journal of alcohol and drug education, 30(2), 12-23.

Suggestions are made for educational program development that includes the fostering of self-esteem, challenges the student out of boredom, creates a climate of involved community, positively influences the direction of the peer culture, exposes the student to wide varieties of experience, fosters the development of personal morality and values, and teaches that stress management will be the most effective in prevention efforts.

446. Horan, J., and Williams, J. (1982). Longitudinal study of assertion training as a drug abuse prevention strategy. American educational research journal, 19(3), 341-351.

Assesses the effects of assertiveness training with junior high school students as a drug prevention effort. After three years, students who had received the training demonstrated increased assertive behaviors and less drug-related behavior.

447. Iverson, D. (1978). Utilizing a health behavior model to design drug education/prevention programs. Journal of drug education, 8(4), 279-287.

Discusses the need to design prevention programs from a health behavior model. The Health Belief Model is proposed as the model of choice.

* Johnson, N. (1982). Michigan develops curriculum to reduce DWI among youth. Alcohol, health and research world, 7(1), 35-37.

See No. 241.

* Kentucky Department of Education, Bureau of Instruction. (1980). Making decisions: Alcohol and drug education guide K-12. Frankfort, KY: Author.

See No. 247.

* Kinard, B. (1982). 97th Congress, February 1982, Testimony of Beverly J. Kinard, In:

Hearing ... Ninety-Seventh Congress. Salt Lake City, UT: Utah Congress of Parents and Teachers.

See No. 255.

448. Kline, J., and Wilson, W. (1972). Ex-addicts in drug abuse prevention education. Drug forum, 1(4), 3357-366.

Describes a prevention program designed and implemented by ex-addicts. It used macropresentations and small group encounters. Students and teachers both responded well to the presentation. Major criticisms were that the ex-addicts failed to make clear the differences between use and abuse and the differences between various psychotropic drugs.

* Kopita, R. (1973). Searchlight: Relevant resources in high interest areas. 4U update search. Counseling for drug abuse. Ann Arbor, MI: ERIC Clearinghouse on Counseling and Personnel Services.

See No. 291.

449. Krupka, L., and Knox, L. (1985). Enhancing the effectiveness of alcohol and substance abuse prevention programs for children. International journal of the addictions, 20(9), 1435-1442.

Tested the hypothesis that exposure to substance abusers in treatment would alter the attitudes and knowledge of a group of eighth grade students. The conclusions indicated that intensive education prevention efforts of this nature are appropriate for this age group and that the experience enhanced the prevention efforts as it related to this group of students.

450. Landress, H. (1983). School-based prevention program for potential drug abusers. Social work in education, 5(4), 241-257.

Describes the development of a prevention program geared towards high risk students in grades three, four, and five. It requires the involvement of both parent and teacher. The students attend the prevention program three days a week and attend their regular school for the remaining days. The program is designed on a "token" economy system with points being earned for good, positive behaviors. In addition, they attend group and individual counseling. No evaluation information is provided.

* Lassey, M., and Carlson, J. (1981). Teenage drinking in Idaho's rural communities. Moscow, ID: University of Idaho College of Agriculture.

See No. 110.

451. Luksetich, W. (1975). The economics of crime: A teaching unit for grades 7-12. St. Cloud, MN: Saint Cloud State College, Center for Economic Education.

Describes a teaching guide for grades 7-12 that relates economic principles and reasoning to an analysis of the causes and remedies of crime.

* Malvin, J., and others. (1985). Evaluation of two school-based alternative programs. Journal of alcohol and drug education, 30(3), 98-108.

See No. 275.

452. Malvin, J., Moskowitz, J., Schaeffer, G., and Schaps, E. (1984). Teacher training in affective education for the primary prevention of adolescent drug abuse. American journal of drug and alcohol abuse, 10(2), 223-235.

Evaluates two student groups: the first taught by teachers trained in a "generic" primary prevention program, the second taught by teachers with more conventional training.

The first group was expected to benefit from this exposure by adopting more positive attitudes, behaviors, and norms in regard to themselves, peers, teachers, and school. Results indicate that for males there was a pattern of negative treatment effects and for females there was no evident treatment effect. Further discussion is given on problems inherent in this type of strategy for adolescent substance abuse prevention.

453. Martin, W. (1972). Operation Drug Prevention: A curriculum guide K-12. Pensacola, FL: University of West Florida.

Describes a K-12 sequential curriculum guide program in drug prevention that was developed for teachers. It is written in outline style and organized according to three areas: content, suggested student activities, and resources and materials. Appendixes are included for reference.

* Mason, V. and Baker, G. (1978). Growing up and feeling powerful as an American Indian. Rockville, MD: National Institute on Drug Abuse.

See No. 278.

454. Massachusetts State Department of Education. (1971). Health education curriculum guide, Grades 1-12. Boston, MA: Author.

Developed to assist local school districts develop stronger, more effective, school health programs. The guide is broken into four broad categories of health education. Each is followed by suggested curriculum for the various grade levels.

455. Mazza, N. (1979). Poetry: A therapeutic tool in the early stages of alcoholism treatment. Journal of studies on alcohol, 40(1), 123-128.

Examines the use of poetry as a therapeutic tool in the initial stages of treatment for alcoholism. Presents methods of using poetry in individual and group methods. Case histories of using poetry with alcoholics and drug abusers are presented.

* Mental Health Materials Center. A selective guide to audiovisuals for mental health and family life education. (1979). Chicago, IL: Marquis Academic Media.

See No. 578.

* Mental Health Materials Center. A selective guide to audiovisuals for mental health and family life education. (1979). Chicago, IL: Marquis Academic Media.

See No. 579.

456. McAlister, A. (1983). Social-psychological approaches. National Institute on Drug Abuse: Research monograph series, 47, 36-50.

Evaluates a prevention effort to prevent adolescent abuse of tobacco through a social-psychological process. Five schools were involved. Findings conclude that friends' smoking habits were more influential on students who had poor relations with their families than students who were close to their parents or teachers. Findings do not support the belief that self-image plays an indirect role in the onset of smoking but that alienation from parents and teachers is an indirect influence toward smoking.

457. McClellan, P. (1975). The Pulaski Project: An innovative drug abuse prevention program in an urban high school. Journal of psychedelic drugs, 7(4), 355-362.

Describes a school-based prevention program which consists of an "alternative class" for drug abusers, discussion in regular classes, long-range training of a volunteer group, and a referral mechanism. The class emphasized exploration of new experiences by nonchemical methods, such as encounter, meditation, and chanting. The program reports reducing the usage of drugs, particularly barbiturates, amphetamines, and psychedelics, but notes an increase in alcohol usage.

* Mills, K. and McCarty, D. (1983). A data based alcohol abuse prevention program in a university setting. Journal of alcohol and drug education, 28(2), 15-27.

See No. 114.

* Mills, K., Neal, E., and Peed-Neal, I. (1983). Handbook for alcohol education: The community approach. Cambridge, MA: Ballinger.

See No. 283.

458. Missouri State Department of Education. (1975). Improvement through innovation. Jefferson City, MO: Author.

Describes 45 ESA Title III programs offered in Missouri. Among other topics are drug and alcohol prevention program curricula.

459. Mitchel, M., Hu, T., McDonnell, N., and Swisher, J. (1984). Cost effectiveness analysis of an educational drug abuse prevention program. Journal of drug education, 14(3), 271-292.

Evaluated cost-effectiveness of three drug abuse prevention curricula programs: religion, health, and social studies. It was found that the religion-based program had more desirable effects on drug abuse prevention and was more cost-effective.

460. Moskowitz, J. (1985). Evaluating the effects of parent groups on the correlates of adolescent substance abusers. Journal of psychoactive drugs, 17(3), 173-178.

Investigates the effect that parent groups have on influencing positive changes in student substance abuse and its correlates.

This was done through interviews with various school personnel and examination of school records. The following correlates were examined: student achievement, absenteeism, vandalism, discipline problems, and course enrollment. Reductions in marijuana use on campus and improvements in class attendance were noted by school personnel. School records were inadequate to document reported changes in student behavior. Factors suggest that retrospective investigations are inadequate for evaluating the stated hypothesis.

461. Moskowitz, J. (1983). Preventing adolescent substance abuse through drug education. Rockville, MD: National Institute on Drug Abuse. Research monograph series, 47, 36-50.

Examines drug education as a preventive solution to the problem of abuse of alcohol, cigarettes, and psychoactive drugs. It further examines the theoretical basis for these programs and the relevancy of these to the problem. The author contends that there is little evidence that adolescent abuse of substances is related to the theoretical underpinnings of these programs or that education alone will not prevent the emergence of substance abuse problems.

* Moskowitz, J., Malvin, J., Schaeffer, G., and Schaps, E. (1983). Evaluation of a junior high school primary prevention program. Addictive behaviors, 8(4), 393-401.

See No. 289.

* Moskowitz, J., Schaps, E., Schaeffer, G., and Malvin, J. (1984). Evaluation of a substance abuse prevention program for junior high school students. International journal of the addictions, 19(4), 419-430.

See No. 290.

* Myers, E. (1973). Applying a Casual Approach to Drug Education. Journal of drug education, 3(4), 415-418.

See No. 12.

462. National Association of Independent Insurers. (1982). Driving alcohol and other drugs off the road. Des Plaines, IL: Author.

Presents materials concerning drinking and driving among teenagers and strategies for discussing the reasons to discuss their drinking and driving.

463. National Coordinating Council on Drug Education. (1975). Super Me/Super You. A bilingual activity book for young children and guide for parents, teachers, and older brothers and sisters. Washington, DC: Author.

Written to develop cognitive and emotional skills in young children to prevent drug abuse. The book offers activities and stories in Spanish and English which are intended to give children a sense of accomplishment, help them in making choices, teach them to understand, and express their feelings. Recommendations for additional readings are made.

464. National Diffusion Network. (1986). Educational Programs That Work--Edition 12. Longmont, CA: Sopris West, Inc.

Presents alternative school-based programs that are based on curriculum and teaching strategies. Curricula are described that address all subject areas in addition to drug and alcohol prevention materials through effective education. Pre-service and in-service education programs are described.

465. National Institute on Drug Abuse. (1981). Saying No--Drug Abuse prevention ideas for the classrooom. Rockville, MD: Author.

Presents a variety of activities, materials, teacher strategies, and other relevant materials for classroom prevention programs. Suggestions for teachers and teaching styles are made. No specific grade levels are addressed and it is implied that all materials can be adjusted for all grade levels.

466. National Institute on Drug Abuse. (1982). Teaching tools for primary prevention: A guide to classroom curricula. Rockville, MD: Author.

Presents a review of materials that are presently being used in various school districts throughout the United States at all grade levels. The guide describes and lists them by age/grade level for different student groups. Information is available on sources of materials and whatever costs may be involved.

* National Institute of Mental Health. (1971). A Guide to drug abuse education and information materials. Chevy Chase, MD: National Clearinghouse for Drug Abuse Information.

See No. 295.

467. New York State Department of Education. (1982). Drug education curriculum--Senior high school. Albany, NY: Author.

Describes the curricula offered in New York State schools for drug abuse, use education. Contains curriculum, suggested teaching methods, classroom activities, learning objectives, and a topical outline for a drug education curriculum. Appended are definitions of drug abuse prevention, materials for minority students, a list of relevant periodicals, a suggested bibliography for parents, references for school staff, and a list of signs of drug use and misuse. This is part of a series that addresses other grade levels.

468. New York State Department of Education. (1986). Health education syllabus--Grades K-12. Albany, NY: Author.

Presents health education curricula and includes drug abuse and alcohol abuse education prevention materials. All subjects are outlined by concepts, instructional objectives, program components, instructional guides, and recommended learner outcomes. An evaluation guide is suggested for individual and program outcomes.

* New York State--Division of Alcoholism and Alcohol Abuse. Fetal alcohol syndrome. (1979). New York: Author.

See No. 49.

469. New York State Education Department. (1976). Alcohol education: A teacher's curriculum guide for grades K-6. Albany, NY: Author.

Presents a curriculum guide for grades K-6. Covers the following areas: Why alcohol education is important, what should be taught, how alcohol education should be taught. Includes supplementary content information for the teacher as well as a resource list for use by the teacher. This is one of a series of three guides which includes, in addition to K-6, guides suitable for 7-12, and adult education.

470. New York Education Department. (1976). Alcohol education: Curriculum guide for grades K-6. Albany, NY: Author.

Designed to assist school personnel in more effective ways to combat the alcohol problem through education as a primary prevention vehicle. Practice experiences comprise the most important components of the elementary education curriculum for decision-making. Each section is divided into separate grade levels identifying topics and the related objective.

* Norem-Hebeisen, A., Ardyth, A., and Lucas, M. (1977). A developmental model for primary prevention of chemical abuse. Journal of drug education, 7(2), 141-148.

See No. 123.

* Nortoft, B., and Dorn, N. (1982). Health careers: Teachers' manual. London, England: Institute for the Study of Drug Dependence.

See No. 51.

471. Nowlis, H. (1976). Strategies for prevention. Contemporary drug problems, 5(1), 5-20.

Describes four models of prevention programs and the processes they employ. These include legal, medical, psychosocial, and sociocultural programs. Objectives of drug education are listed and described.

* Nowlis, H. (1977). Statement before the Subcommittee on Alcoholism and Drug Abuse, Committee on Human Resources, United States Senate. Washington, DC: United States Government Printing Office.

See No. 609.

* Nowlis, H. (1980, March). Prevention is not easy. Paper presented at the First Pan-Pacific Conference on Drugs and Alcohol, Canberra, Australia, March.

See No. 610.

472. Olton, A. (1985). The effect of locus of control and perceptions of school environment on outcome in three school drug abuse prevention programs. Journal of drug education, 15(2), 157-169.

Investigated the effects of student locus of control and their perceptions of school environment as it related to their outcome in an alternative school-based drug abuse prevention program. Scores on the Norwicki-Strickland Locus of Control Scale were significant in the multivariate analysis. Certain interactions between locus of control and school perceptions affected some of the outcome variables.

473. Pepperman, C. (1982). Supporting humanistic learning. Humanist educator, 20(4), 187-192.

Defends the humanistic learning theories for drug prevention programs. In addition, responses are provided for the back-to-basics critics as well as those who label this method as trendy.

474. Philadelphia School District. (1980). Key competencies: Drug and alcohol education. Elementary schools. Philadelphia, PA: Author.

Describes educational prevention programs designed for use with elementary school students. Presents curriculum materials, activities, and learning objectives designed to increase self-esteem, enhance self-image, develop values, and enable children to develop identities.

* Pringle, H., Gregory, J., Ginkel, K., and Cheek, C. (1981). Alpha centers: A viable prevention model for substance abuse agencies and public schools. In: A. J. Schecter (Ed.), Drug dependency and alcoholism, Vol. 2: Social behavior issues. New York, NY: Plenum Press.

See No. 126.

475. Ramsey, E. (1982). An intervention model for alcohol and drug problems on college campuses. Journal of college student personnel, 23(4), 346-348.

Describes the development and implementation of the Chemical Use Abuse Group Program, an educational program designed to prevent chemical abuse and to motivate students with chemical abuse problems to seek appropriate treatment.

476. Reynolds, J.C., and Wootton, L.R. (1972). Health education: Golden opportunity for the middle school. Clearinghouse, 47(4), 219-222.

Describes a carefully planned health education curriculum that aids in overcoming seven health problems including drug and alcohol abuse.

477. Ryan, W., and Hettena, C. (1976). Project youth: An approach to drug abuse. Elementary school guidance and counseling, 10(4), 270-278.

Describes a school-based program offered in the New York City school system. It is composed of a professional trained in group work and a paraprofessional who is a community resident and has had some college training. The program consists of groups that are co-led and focus on structured and unstructured tasks. In addition, groups are offered for parents of students.

* Safford, P., Deighan, W., Corder, L., and Miller, W. (1975). Training teachers for drug abuse prevention: A humanistic approach. Journal of drug education, 5(4), 355-349.

See No. 57.

* Sexter, J., Sullivan, A., Wepner, S., and Denmark, R. (1984). Substance abuse: Assessment of the outcomes of activities and activity clusters in school-based prevention. International journal of the addictions, 19(1), 79-92.

See No. 331.

478. Sheppard, M. (1984). Drug abuse prevention education: What is realistic for schools? Journal of drug education, 14(4), 323-329.

Discusses various issues in drug use and abuse to explore how preventive drug abuse measures in schools could address these issues. Potential school-based interventions are described.

479. Simmons, R. (1973). An alternative curriculum model for urban education and community

affairs programs in higher education. Wayne, NJ: William Paterson College, Department of Urban Education.

Describes the urban education program which is defined as educating people for living and coping with an urban environment, including drug and alcohol abuse.

480. Stenmark, D., Walfish, S., and Brennan, A. (1981). A three course sequence in substance abuse prevention at the baccalaureate level. Teaching of psychology, 8(2), 82-85.

The courses included an overview of the substance abuse field, a skill building course in substance abuse prevention, and a practicum for hands-on experience in the field of substance abuse.

481. Stoessel, R. (1974). The school system ought to assume a creative role. CEMEF informa, 2(3), 14-15.

Asserts that to solve the problem of drug abuse by students, school systems must adopt a creative role in developing ethical values in children. The author contends that it is not enough to foster intellectual and academic development, emotional and social development must also be promoted.

482. Swanson, J. (1978). The "no win": Drug education evaluation problems. Journal of drug education, 8(2), 125-129.

Suggests that confusion of the goals of prevention and treatment have led some schools to define the goals of their drug abuse education programs so that they cannot reasonably achieve success. Concludes that a new model of evaluation for such goals has to be developed.

483. Swisher, J., and Hu, T. (1983). Alternatives to drug abuse: Some are and some are not. National Institute on Drug Abuse: Research monograph series, 47, 141-153.

Evaluates and reviews current prevention efforts. Describes four models of alternative programming for prevention efforts. These include specific activities for youth, matching types of needs with types of activities, reinforcing participation in existing alternate activities, and facilitating youth-directed groups in the process of initiating self-selected activities. Suggests that more longitudinal research on underlying psychosocial dynamics needs to be conducted regarding the behavioral manifestations of substance abuse and prevention.

484. Swisher, J., Nesselroade, C., and Tatanish, C. (1985). Here's Looking at You Two is looking good: An experimental analysis. Journal of humanistic education and development, 23(3), 111-119.

Evaluates a humanistically-based alcohol and drug education curriculum titled "Here's Looking at You Two." Findings show that use of tobacco, marijuana, and stimulants was significantly lower among students who had been exposed to the curriculum. Results were nearly significant for depressants and alcohol. Suggests strong support for a carefully designed and implemented affective/humanistic approach to substance abuse prevention.

485. Taylor, W. (1974). Touching lives: Pattern of healthful living, Level 4. A values curriculum, Second revision. Harris County Department of Education: Houston, TX.

Contains value-based curriculum lessons which are intended to assist students in the development of positive self-concept, rational thinking processes, inter- and intra-personal skills, and a personal and social values system. Suggests teaching techniques which include readings, classroom discussions, use of filmstrips, games, and interviews. Each suggested lesson outline contains purpose, concepts, affective objectives, classroom activities, teaching procedures, guiding questions, evaluation techniques, and lists of materials needed.

486. Texas Education Agency, Austin Division of Crime Prevention and Drug Education. (1975). Administrators' handbook for crime prevention and drug education. Austin, TX: Author.

Describes a program for crime prevention in school systems that has been mandated by the Texas State Legislature. To be included in all grades from K-12.

487. Texas Education Agency. (1971). Elementary school health curriculum guide. Austin, TX: Author.

Presents a comprehensive health education program for grades K-6. It is designed to promote discussion and build concepts rather than to give specific information. Each area is divided into two levels, primary and intermediate, and outlines the major concept, subconcepts, behavioral objectives, content, motivating questions, and suggested learning experiences. Materials and their sources are appended.

488. Texas Education Agency. (1971). Secondary school health curriculum guide. Austin, TX: Author.

Presents a comprehensive health education program for grades 7-12. It is designed to promote discussion and build concepts rather than to give specific information. Each area is divided into two levels, primary and intermediate, and outlines the major concept, subconcepts, behavioral objectives, content, motivating questions, and suggested learning experiences. Materials, bibliography, learning activities, and their sources are appended.

489. Torrence, W., and Hanna, M. (1981). Administrative planning for a fusion of systems: Where prevention and treatment must merge. In: A.J. Schecter, (Ed.), Drug dependence and alcoholism. Vol. 2: Social behavior issues. New York, NY: Plenum Press.

Presents a model curriculum and a program process designed specifically for youth who may be experiencing sufficient drug or alcohol problems as to warrant a full time residential program. The components of the program are presented and the benefits of a holistic approach for treatment, as well as for prevention and education, are discussed.

490. United States Jaycees. (1975). All in the family: Understanding how we teach and influence children about alcohol. Participants' workbook and chairman's guide. Tulsa, OK: Author.

Describes a program offered by the Jaycees called Operation THRESHOLD. The material focuses primarily on prevention through small group discussion to elicit responses on how we teach and influence children. Useful as a parent/child guide or as a participant's workbook in an informal group setting.

491. Wayne County Intermediate School District. (1971). Values clarification (Decisions, drugs, values). Lansing, MI: Michigan State Department of Education.

Presents a how-to-do-it booklet for teachers on how to use values clarification in drug education.

492. Webb, R., Egger, G., and Reynolds, I. (1978). Prediction and prevention of drug abuse. Journal of drug education, 8(3), 221-230.

Describes prevention efforts from an infectious disease model. This is a follow up to a previous paper where the characteristics of the potential addict are described. Reports of productive and counterproductive educational techniques based on research findings and international reports on the outcomes of effective and counterproductive programs are included.

493. Weisheit, R. (1984). Alcohol and drug abuse prevention: Implications for delinquency

prevention. Journal of drug issues, 14(3), 469-477.

Argues that drug and alcohol education programs may provide important information regarding delinquency prevention. It is suggested that these programs can also provide data relative to the link between alcohol/drugs and delinquency, as well as the implementation of school-based primary delinquency prevention programs. The problems of developing and implementing delinquency prevention programs are reviewed.

* Winn, M. (1974). The drug alternative. Washington, DC: American Alliance for Health, Physical Education, and Recreation.

See No. 523.

* Worick, W., and Schaller, W. (1977). Alcohol, tobacco, and drugs: Their use and abuse. Englewood Cliffs, NJ: Prentice-Hall.

See No. 524.

494. Zoller, U. and Weiss, S. (1981). "Hashish and Marijuana"--An innovative, interdisciplinary drug education curriculum program for high schools. Journal of drug education, 11(1), 37-43.

Describes a preventive education program developed for schools in Israel. It is described as an appropriate model for implementation within the realm of natural and social science courses. It equally emphasizes the cognitive and affective domains. The authors indicate that the curriculum was favorably accepted by students and research findings indicate good results.

LEARNING PERFORMANCE

495. Bustamente, J., et al. (1969). Learning and drugs. Revista interamericana de psicologia, 3(2), 67-82.

Presents the findings of a study with 810 students to determine what effects amphetamines and barbiturates have on learning nonsense syllables. The results suggest that what is learned at a determined level drops when the level changes and tends to reestablish itself upon return to the original level.

496. Conners, C. (1969). A teacher rating scale for use in drug studies with children. American journal of psychiatry, 126(6), 884-888.

Describes and emphasizes the value of a symptom and behavior rating checklist for teachers' use in drug studies with children. A treatment study of dextroamphetamine with a group of children having learning and/or behavior disorders showed significant changes in all factors compared with a placebo group in a double blind study.

497. Hurst, P., Radlow, R., Chubb, N., and Bagley, S. (1969). Effects of d-amphetamine on acquisition, persistence and recall. American journal of psychology, 82(3), 307-319.

Presents the findings of a study that measured the effects of d-amphetamine in a paired associate learning task. 69 male undergraduates were tested in two sessions, for learning and delayed recall. Findings indicate that presence of d-amphetamine during learning recall resulted in significantly greater delayed recall of the low competition lists and nonsignificantly greater delayed recall of high competition lists. The same dose given for the recall session had no significant effect upon delayed recall or relearning.

498. Lewis, E., Dustman, R., and Beck, E. (1969). The effect of alcohol on sensory phenomenon and cognitive and motor tasks. Quarterly journal of studies on alcohol, 30(3-A), 618-633.

Presents the findings of a study that evaluated the effects of alcohol on motor task and memory. Four sensory and four cognitive and motor tasks were administered to ten male moderate drinkers after alcohol and placebo consumption. The absence of alcoholic effect on the majority of the tasks is discussed in terms of the brevity of each task, practice effects, and compensation.

* Sieber, J., and others. (1976). The effects of learning when to be uncertain on children's knowledge and use of drugs. R and D memorandum No. 144. Stanford, CA: Stanford University, Center for Research and Development in Teaching.

See No. 333.

PREVENTION PROGRAMS

Community Based

499. American Institue for Research in the Behavioral Sciences. (1970). <u>Police youth protection unit programs, San Jose, California: Model programs, Childhood education</u>. Palo Alto, CA: Author.

Describes a prevention program developed and implemented by the Palo Alto Police Department. It has as its goal, in addition to drug abuse prevention, general delinquency prevention, etc.

500. Aubrey, R. (1971). School-Community drug prevention programs. <u>Personnel and guidance journal</u>, <u>50</u>(1), 17-24.

Presents a ten-point program for schools and communities. The program's thrust is an endeavor whereby key individuals and agencies in the community are involved in long range efforts to dissuade youngsters from harmful experimentation with drugs.

* Anastas, R. (1982, August). <u>Prepared statement for the U.S. Senate Committee on Alcoholism and Drug Abuse</u>. U.S. Senate Hearing on Alcohol, Drugs and Driving. Washington, DC: United States Government Printing Office.

See No. 150.

* Clements, M. (1978). Health and drug education--A regional approach. <u>Educational leadership</u>, <u>35</u>(4), 314-317.

See No. 435.

* Cohen, A. (1973). Alternatives to drug abuse: Steps towards prevention. Rockville, MD: National Institute on Drug Abuse.

See No. 86.

501. Coleman, J. (1978). Deviant subcultures and the schools. In: Theoretical perspectives on school crime. Vol. I. Washington, DC: Department of Health, Education and Welfare.

Describes typical school crimes, drug abuse, vandalism, and theft, as phenomena of subcultures, groups that have different sets of values, attitudes, and perspectives. Several recommendations for school policy are made on the basis of subcultural theory, including the restructuring of educational institutions to reduce student alienation and status deprivation and the creation of programs to encourage involvement in nondeviant subcultures.

* Coleman, S. (1978). Sib group therapy: A prevention program for siblings from drug addicted families. International journal of the addictions, 13(1), 115-127.

See No. 526.

* Dembo, R., and Miran, M. (1975). Evaluation of drug prevention programs by youths in a middle class community. International journal of the addictions, 11(5).

See No. 92.

* Dembo, R., Schmeidler, J., Taylor, R., and Burgos, W. (1982). Supports for, and consequences of, early drug involvement among inner city junior high school youths living in three neighborhood settings. Journal of drug education, 12(3), 191-210.

See No. 380.

* Dickinson, L., and others. (1973). A comparison of three community drug abuse

programs including clientele, cost, and effectiveness. Journal of drug education, 3(3), 247-259.

See No. 195.

* Eiseman, S. (1974). An approach to primary prevention of drug abuse among children and youth-parental influence. Journal of drug education, 4(1), 27-35.

See No. 572.

502. Gordon, P. (1971). Approaches to drug abuse prevention. Journal of drug education, 1(3), 275-277.

Describes the drug abuse related definitions of the words education and prevention. The author contends that the changing use of these terms is an indication of the enlightened approach to ameliorating the problem of drug abuse.

* Hewitt, L. (1982). Current status of alcohol education programs for youth. In: Alcohol and health mono. no. 4: Special populations. Washington, DC: United States Government Printing Office.

See No. 102.

503. Horan, J. (1973). Preventing drug abuse through behavior change technology. Journal of Student Personnel Association for Teacher Education, 11(4), 145-152.

Describes several aspects of behavioral learning theory and shows how they can be applied to the understanding of drug abuse with illustrations of their role in behavioral group counseling, a promising new strategy for drug abuse prevention.

504. Imhoff, J. and others. (1972). The emerging role of the hospital in drug abuse education and prevention. Journal of school health, 42(8), 472-476.

Describes the role the hospital can play in the prevention of drug abuse through involvement within the schools. Further indicates that the hospital can provide education and training programs for those working with drug-involved individuals.

505. Jacobs, P. (1977). A rural response to drug abuse. Paper revised for the Rural Sociological Society Meeting, Madison, WI.

Describes the efforts of rural Pike county, Ohio's efforts to combat drug abuse. The program includes primary and secondary efforts, i.e., drug education to schools and community; individual, group and family counseling; criminal justice referrals/intakes; drug diversion/prevention; crisis intervention. The paper focuses prevention efforts at the development of quality interpersonal skill building.

* Jacobson, M. (1983, January). Parent movement in the United States. Paper presented at the Tenth Biennial Summer School of the National Society on Alcoholism and Drug Dependency, Wellington, New Zealand.

See No. 577.

* Kaiser, L. (Ed.). (1983). Chemical people book. Pittsburgh, PA: QED Enterprises.

See No. 105.

506. Kaminsky, K. (1978). Affective education: A positive approach to school crime. In: Theoretical Perspectives on School Crime. Vol. I. Washington, DC: Department of Health, Education and Welfare.

Presents theoretical data on the role of affective education in lowering school crime and drug use in school. The theories presented are based on quality educational efforts, i.e., Schools Without Failure and Values Clarification.

507. Laria, J. (1971). Drug education and prevention: A human relations and school community approach. National Catholic Guidance Conference journal, 15(4), 262-265.

Describes a prevention effort that is built upon a human relations model.

* Larsen, B., Krynak, D., and Pettyjohn, T. (1981). Alcohol and other drug use among rural adolescents: Some implications for rural drug programming. In: A.J. Schecter (Ed.), Drug dependency and alcoholism, Vol. 2: Social behavior issues. New York, NY: Plenum Press

See No. 109.

508. Loers, D., and Sarata, B. (1983, August). A community development model for prevention of chemical abuse. Paper presented at the Annual Convention of the American Psychological Association, Anaheim, CA.

Describes the efforts of the rural Pioneer Mental Health Center, Seward, Nebraska. The development of the program is described in detail. The authors stress process oriented activities to promote a sense of community. The effect of this type of orientation is discussed. Useful for anyone planning to develop a community-based prevention program.

509. National Drug Center for Training and Resource Development. (1981). Community based prevention specialist, trainer manual. Washington, DC: Author.

Presents a trainer's manual designed to assist facilitators in the design of entry-level courses and programs for substance abuse prevention specialist.

* National Institute on Alcohol Abuse and Alcoholism. (1984). Prevention plus: Involving schools, parents, and the community in alcohol and drug education. Rockville, MD: Author.

See No. 13.

510. Palais, E. (1973). Drug abuse treatment: The cart before the horse. Journal of drug education, 3(2), 153-155.

Assesses the financial resources made available to treatment programs versus prevention programs. The author contends that it is time to look at the problem in its proper perspective, namely prevention and a willingness on the part of some of us to admit it exists.

511. Pearson, J. (1971). Juvenile drug abuse prevention project. First year program evaluation. Washington, DC: National Institute of Law Enforcement and Criminal Justice.

Describes a program whose intention was to divert court processing of a large number of adolescents with no apparent increase in risk. Included is a brief description of the background review of the development of the program, research activities and methods, and discussion relating to each of the grant proposal objectives.

* Recchia, C. (1982, April 4). Treating youthful alcoholics. News-American, Baltimore, MD.

See No. 398.

* Schuchard, M. (1982). National parents' movement for drug free youth. In: PRIDE Southeast Drug Conference Proceedings, 1980 and 1981. Atlanta, GA: PRIDE.

See No. 326.

512. Slawson, M., and Kopacz, K. (1972). Community involvement in prevention and control of drug abuse. Journal of drug education, 2(2), 139-147.

Emphasizes the need for community involvement and responsibility in controlling drug abuse. Illustrates this through the description of the New York State legislation that gave rise to the Narcotic Guidance Councils. These Councils provided prevention education, secondary prevention efforts to individuals and their families, as well as treatment.

* Social Advocates for Youth. (1978). Early age prevention of alcohol abuse project: Final report. San Francisco, CA: Author.

See No. 134.

513. Solis, J., and Johnson, C. (1983). Comprehensive community programs for drug abuse implications of the Community Heart Disease Prevention Programs for future research. In: Preventing adolescent drug abuse: Intervention strategies. Rockville, MD: National Institute on Drug Abuse.

Explores the prevention of drug and alcohol abuse, as well as cigarette smoking, in an entire community. Discusses some current community prevention projects and the evaluations conducted simultaneously. Recommendations for future research in community prevention projects are made.

* Stolz, P., and Van Der Heide, G. (1983, May). School/Community intervention workshop: A workshop on the CADAP (Community Alcohol and Drug Abuse Prevention). Paper presented at the National Drug Institute, Brisbane, Australia.

See No. 23.

514. Sugarman, B. (1978). Drug abuse prevention: A human development model for defining the problem and devising solutions. Drug forum: The journal of human issues, 6(4), 387-397.

Describes drug abuse as a deficit in the human development process, as one of several behavior patterns with which the individual attempts to fill an "emotional vacuum." Notes that effective drug abuse prevention must involve the improvement of the environment. Distinctions between primary prevention, secondary prevention, and rehabilitation are made.

515. Thorsheim, H., and Roberts, B. (1983). The "Flavor" of the social ecology paradigm in use: Building on mutual social support in prevailing drug abuse. Paper presented at the Annual Convention of the American Psychological Association, Anaheim, CA.

Describes a community prevention program that is based on a social ecology theory. The program intends to prevent drug abuse through the development of socially supportive relationships and through using the environment as a natural strength within the community.

* Ventura, M., and Dundon, M. (1974). A challenging experience in canoeing and camping as a tool in approaching the drug problem. Journal of drug education, 4(1), 123-127.

See No. 361.

516. Volpe, R. (1977). Feedback facilitated relaxation training as primary prevention of drug abuse in early adolescence. Journal of drug education, 7(2), 179-189.

Describes the use of relaxation training as a means of primary prevention to develop self-esteem and to reduce drug abuse. The aim of this paper is to provide an overview of relaxation training and electromyography and to focus this approach on the needs of early adolescents.

* West, P., and others. (1976). Report on a needs assessment and evaluation of a drug education program. Van Nuys, CA: Los Angeles Valley College.

See No. 369.

* Wilson, W., and Helm, S. (1970). An alcoholism program tailored to community

needs. Hospital and community psychiatry, 21(12), 406-408.

See No. 66.

517. Wolfe, H., and Haynes, D. (1973). State-Local partnership against addiction: A report on a drug education-prevention pilot project in metropolitan New York. (1973). Journal of drug education, 3(2), 189-200.

Describes a project that was funded by the New York State Department of Mental Hygiene in 1969-1970 at a cost of $400,000. Its primary emphasis was on dealing with drug-related social and economic problems and finding alternatives to drug abuse.

Multi-Stage Models

518. American Automobile Association. (1976). You ... Alcohol and driving. (DOOT-HS-5-01195). Washington, DC: National Highway Traffic Safety Administration.

 Presents a complete and comprehensive look at drinking while under the influence of drugs or alcohol. Keyed to the "If you drive, what about alcohol?" series.

519. Bedworth, D. (1971). Approaches to drug abuse prevention: Crusade vs. fact of life. Journal of drug education, 1(3), 285-291.

 Presents some suggestions for dealing with the problem of adequately utilizing the educational resources available in preparing students to cope with the problems they will face in a drug-oriented society.

520. Creighton, H. (1975). Health education encounters. New York: J. Wiley & Sons.

 Describes a program whereby students learn self-knowledge and understanding of physical needs, safety, sexuality, health services, products, and disease prevention for themselves and others. This book focuses on certain aspects of growth and health: emotions, personality, social behavior, sexual development, sexual consideration and responsibility, the difficulties and rewards of having friends, and the constant adjustments required to maintain worthwhile relations with other people. A guide for teachers is available. Suggests that through proper education and development the risk of drug usage is lessened.

* Shields, E., and others. (1973, March). Choicepoint: A peer group model for facilitating decision making. Paper presented at the American College Personnel Association, Atlanta, GA.

See No. 21.

521. Smith, C. (1971). Drug education: Reasons and failures. Journal of drug education, 1(4), 373-389.

Presents 50 reasons why drug abuse continues to increase. These reasons are grouped into ten categories. The author concludes that educational programs that are built on simplistic cause models are relatively ineffective. Further, the author concludes that honest education is necessary.

* Swisher, J., and others. (1973). Four approaches to drug abuse prevention among college students. Journal of college student personnel, 13(3), 231-235.

See No. 139.

* U.S. Department of Health and Human Services. (1981). The Door: A model youth center. Rockville, MD: Author.

See No. 358.

522. Voas, R. (1974). Alcohol, drugs and young drivers. Washington, DC: National Highway Traffic Safety Administration.

Reviews the literature available on the relationship of drugs, alcohol, and a group of young criminals. The data suggest that young people use drugs more than adults do, and that they drive more often under the influence of drugs and alcohol--more often than adults do, consequently young people are more vulnerable to accidents than the adult groups. The author suggests various countermeasures to offset this. The author concludes that few countermeasures, to date, have demonstrated effectiveness. Nevertheless, he argues that it is essential for more effort to be placed in this direction.

523. Winn, M. (1974). The drug alternative. Washington, DC: American Alliance for Health, Physical Education, and Recreation.

Developed for educators and counselors. Contains readings on various developmental aspects that will lead to a choice to remain drug free. Also contains exercises and curriculum modules that can be used in the classroom.

* Wong, M. (1975, April). Different strokes: Models of drug abuse prevention. Paper presented at the Annual Meeting of the American Educational Research Association, Washington, DC.

See No. 372.

524. Worick, W., and Schaller, W. (1977). Alcohol, tobacco, and drugs: Their use and abuse. Englewood Cliffs, NJ: Prentice-Hall.

Examines some of the concerns surrounding drug use and abuse in society. Central to this book is the issue that alcohol, drugs, and tobacco are a part of our society and that our failure to deal with resultant problems is a betrayal of society. Education and prevention are stressed as the ultimate answer, but the authors also recognize that rehabilitation and law enforcement programs must be expanded. Written as a text for college level courses.

FAMILY SYSTEMS

Effects on Prevention

525. Aron, W. (1975). Family background and personal trauma among drug addicts in the United States: Implications for treatment. British journal of addiction, 70(3), 295-305.

Compares data from previous studies with data collected on the characteristics of 346 drug addicts. Conclusions are drawn based on the therapeutic implications of the family disorganization and personal traumas in the backgrounds of the addicts.

526. Coleman, S. (1978). Sib group therapy: A prevention program for siblings from drug addicted families. International journal of the addictions, 13(1), 115-127.

To prevent drug abuse among younger siblings of addicted adolescents, weekly group therapy sessions were implemented at a suburban therapeutic community with fifteen to twenty 10-13 year olds. The concept developed as an outgrowth of family therapy that had revealed that intergernerational addictive patterns might impose a high-risk future of similar behavior among latency age children. Results indicate that severe acting out diminished, but underlying psychodynamics appeared unchanged.

527. Craig, S., and Brown, B. (1975). Comparison of youthful heroin users and nonusers from one urban community. International journal of the addictions, 10(1), 53-64.

Concluded a study of 65 black drug users

participating in a metropolitan drug treatment program and a matched sample of nonusers. Results show that users were significantly less likely than nonusers to have both parents available to them during late childhood; members of drug users' families were significantly more likely to be involved with drugs than members of nonusers' families.

528. Despotovic, A. (1974). Alcoholism, drug addictions and the family. Anali zavoda za mentalno zdravlje, 6(2-3), 191-202.

Reports on the findings of a survey of 757 alcoholics in Belgrade. Studied multiple variables related to family, family structure, etc. These were analyzed with similar data from drug abusers. Suggests that alcoholics can be treated with family therapy techniques. Helpful in understanding the family patterns and characteristics for drug and alcohol abusers.

* Jaynes, J., and Rugg, C. (1983). Role of chemical abuse during adolescence. Focus on alcohol and drug issues, 6(3), 16-17.

See No. 386.

529. Kirschenbaum, M., Leonoff, G., and Maliano, A. (1974). Characteristic patterns in drug abusing families. Family therapy, 1(1), 43-62.

Describes a study of the clinically observable family interaction patterns that characterize families with a drug abusing member. Literature of similar studies is described.

530. Klinge, V., Vaziri, H., and Lennox, K. (1976). Comparison of psychiatric in-patient male and female adolescent drug abusers. International journal of the addictions, 11(2), 309-323.

Presents data from a questionnaire survey

considering etiological, environmental, and social variables. Subjects were 81 male and 62 female drug-abusing adolescent psychiatric in-patients. Results indicated that for females, drug abuse and pathology were associated with family related variables; for males, abuse and pathology emerged as factors inherent to family drug abuse and pathology. The authors conclude that the female addict is more reactive to the family situation and a hypothesis is presented that when a female separates from the family her pathology will decrease more than that of the male who separates.

* Pulkkinen, L. (1982). Smoking and drinking among youth: A longitudinal study. Alkoholipolitiikka, 47(3), 139-146.

See No. 396.

531. Reilly, D. (1975). Family factors in the etiology and treatment of youth drug abuse. Family therapy, 2(2), 149-171.

Describes the use of conjoint family therapy with drug abusers and their families. Steps of the treatment process and therapeutic interventions are described. A profile of the drug-abusing family system is presented and makes suggestions for future research. This project and service can be viewed as a secondary prevention effort.

532. Rollins, J., and Holden, R. (1972). Adolescent drug use and the alienation syndrome. Journal of drug education, 2(3), 249-261.

Reports on adolescent drug use and some of the reasons for it. Research reveals that adolescent drug users are enmeshed in an alienation syndrome and need a variety of services for prevention and rehabilitation.

* Smith, E. (1981). Adolescent drug abuse and alcoholism: Directions for the school and the family. Urban education, 16(3), 311-322.

See No. 336.

533. Stimmel, B. (1975). Factors leading to drug abuse. In B. Stimmel (Ed.). Heroin dependency: Medical, economic and social aspects, New York, NY: Stratton Intercontinental Medical Book Corp.

Summarizes concepts of the characteristics of the male heroin user based on the observations of the authors. Variables centered around the etiology of drug abuse are discussed.

534. Timms, M., Carnyey, P., and Stevenson, R. (1973). A factor analytic study of drug abuse in adolescents. Irish journal of psychology, 2(2), 86-95.

Reports on the findings of a study where the 16PF, Cornell Index, and a demographic and family background questionnaire was administered to 42 male and 8 female 15-25 year old drug users in Dublin, Ireland. It is suggested that the identified classifications are of more use in planning prevention and treatment programs than classifications based on the effects of the drug abused or epidemiological factors.

* Zucker, R., and Noll, R. (1982). Precursors and developmental influences on drinking and etiology from a longitudinal perspective. In: Alcohol and health monograph no. 1: Alcohol consumption and related problems. Washington, DC: Department of Health and Human Services.

See No. 415.

Therapeutic Interventions

535. Amini, F., Sheil, S., and Burke, E. (1976). Adolescent drug abuse: Etiological and treatment considerations. Adolescence, 11(42), 281-299.

Examines the general issues involved in treating adolescent drug abusers, and reviews the literature that describes their personality traits.

536. Aubertin, C. (1968). A pilot project for the treatment of alcoholics: The familial dimension. Tosicomanies, 1(2), 217-219.

Describes a pilot project for the treatment of 71 alcoholics through family therapy as provided by a team of two psychiatrists, one social worker, and one internist.

537. Baither, R. (1978). Family therapy with adolescent drug abusers: A review. Journal of drug education, 8(4), 337-343.

Presents a brief review of the literature, including treatment approaches, processes, goals, and programs. Clear reasons for treating the family of the adolescent drug abuser are discussed.

538. Bartlett, D. (1975). The Use of Multiple Family Therapy Groups with Adolescent Drug Addicts. In: B. Sugar (Ed.), The adolescent in group and family therapy. New York: Brunner/Mazel.

Describes the goals and reasons for treating adolescent drug abusers in both group and family therapy processes. The author expresses concern that all adolescents must be seen in family therapy to truly achieve recovery.

539. Berger, M. (1973). Multifamily psychosocial group treatment with addicts and their families. Group process, 5(1), 31-45.

Describes the narcotic addiction treatment programs of a therapeutic community. Presents and examines the conflicts, attitudes, and disruptive patterns which may have led to drug abuse. Cites the rehabilitative efforts and the etiology of drug abuse.

540. Bieliauskas, V. (1977). Psychology in action: Mental health care in the USSR. American psychologist, 32(5), 376-379.

Desribes how treatment programs in the USSR have begun to use family therapy as a means to treat drug addiction.

541. Bowen, M. (1974). Alcoholism as viewed through family systems theory and family psychotherapy. Annals of the New York Academy of Sciences, 233, 115-122.

Outlines the principles of family systems theory, in which the alcoholism of one member is conceptualized as a symptom of the problem of the larger family or social unit. Cites ways in which systems theory can be used to alleviate these problems.

542. Cahill, T. (1976). The effectiveness of familial involvement on the psychodynamics of adolescent drug user therapy. Dissertation abstracts international, 36(8-B), 4128-4129.

Describes the role of and need for family therapy in the rehabilitation of adolescent drug abusers.

543. Catanzaro, R. (1973). Combined treatment of alcoholics, drug abusers, and related problems in a family residential center. Drug forum, 2(2), 203-212.

Describes and discusses family therapy as an alternative to traditional psychiatric care for persons with alcohol, drug, and personality problems. The central goal of the therapy is to make a person a responsible, caring member of the patient family unit. Upon admission of a member of the natural family, another family member is admitted as a co-patient, the patient learns to transfer his new personality skills into his usual home relationships with the assistance of his natural family member.

544. Coleman, A. (1976). How to enlist the family as an ally. American journal of drug and alcohol abuse, 3(1), 167-173.

Reviews ways that the family of an addict entering a residential treatment program can be enlisted to help in the treatment process. Underscores the role the family of the addict plays in the recovery process.

545. Coleman, S., and Kaplan, D. (1978). A profile of family therapists in the drug abuse field. American journal of drug and alcohol abuse, 5(2), 171-178.

Presents a profile of 1,117 family therapists who were providing treatment to families of recovering drug abusers. Results provide extensive information on the education, training, personal background, caseload characteristics, and theoretical orientations of these therapists.

546. Coleman, S., and Davis, D. (1978). Family therapy and drug abuse: A national survey. Family process, 17(1), 21-29.

Describes a research effort to determine the role of family therapy in 2,012 agencies treating drug abusers with family therapy techniques. A progress index for family therapy programs was developed and used to evaluate 500 agencies. Findings show considerable variation in the expertise, and suggest that methadone maintenance treatment programs had the least sophisticated family therapy treatment.

547. Corenbaum, B., and Fischer, D. (1975). Some correlates of Al-Anon group membership. Journal of studies of alcohol, 36(5), 675-677.

Examines the views of 16 female members of Al-Anon whose husbands were members of the Alcoholic Anonymous program. They indicate that their husbands' association with Alcoholics Anonymous has had positive effects on their roles as father, marital happiness, and problem severity.

548. Davis, D. (1978). Family therapy for the drug user: Conceptual and practical considerations. Drug forum, 6(3), 197-205.

Examines the role of the family in the perpetuation of drug addiction. It further explores the theoretical role of family systems in bringing about total recovery for drug abusers through redesigning the family system of the drug abuser.

549. del Castillo, G., and Grainick, A. (1971). The inpatient treatment of a child drug abuser in a mixed age group. Psychiatric quarterly, 45(4), 593-602.

Presents a case study of a child drug abuser that was refused admission into rehabilitation programs due to his age. He was later admitted into a psychiatric setting where he was treated with adults and adolescents. Recommendations are made for special provisions for drug abusers such as this child. The authors mention some of the etiological factors leading to childhood drug abuse.

550. Dell Orto, A. (1974). The role and resources of the family during the drug rehabilitation process. Journal of psychedelic drugs, 6(4), 435-445.

Reviews problems in the families of drug abusers. In the rehabilitation of addicts, restoration of a "dissonance-free" relation within the family is considered important, but family members may be suffering from emotional strain created by the drug abuser. Therapeutic approaches suggested are family therapy, multifamily therapy, and community involvement.

551. Ferreira, A. (1967). Family therapy in alcoholism. Psychotherapy and psychosomatics, 15(1), 20.

Describes alcoholism as an interactional event. In the husband-wife relationship his (or her) alcoholism is a joint venture that defines the nature of the relationship. Thus, con-joint efforts would seem to be the most reasonable approach to the problem, were it not for the non-acoholic partner who manages to stay out of it. These efforts may have applicability to prevention services with at-risk youth.

552. Fisch, M. (1976). Homeostasis: A key in working with alcoholic families. Family therapy, 3(2), 133-139.

Describes the role of homeostasis in the treatment of alcoholism through family therapy. Case histories are presented to emphasize a systems approach to alcohol treatment.

553. Finlay, D. (1974). Alcoholism: Illness or problem in interaction. Social work, 19(4), 198-405.

Discusses the concept that excessive drinking may be a symptom of a person's faulty interaction with his/her family and significant others. Studies using this social system model are evaluated. Data suggest that rehabilitation workers who viewed alcoholism as an illness did not have as great a success in working with alcoholic patients as did workers who held interaction orientations. Group counseling may be more effective than individual counseling in decreasing drinking. The need for further evaluation of the interactional model is emphasized. Further, limitation of the illness and individualistic models of alcoholism are highlighted.

554. Hagglund, T., and Pylkkanen, K. (1974). Psychotherapy of drug-using adolescent as in-patients and out-patients in a hospital special care unit. Psychiatria fennica, 249-256.

Explores the data reported by 34 in-patient and 152 out-patient drug-abusing clients as well as the data reported by 91 of their families. It is suggested that there is a close relationship between the drug-abusing behaviors and the problems of the entire family.

555. Hendricks, W. (1971). Use of multifamily counseling groups in treatment of male narcotics addicts. International journal of group psychotherapy, 21(1), 84-90.

Describes a study of randomly chosen male drug abusers who participated in multifamily therapy in contrast to those who did not receive family therapy. It is suggested that those who received this form of therapy had a greater success factor in treatment.

556. Hindman, M. (1976). Children of alcoholic parents. Alcohol, health and research world, 2-6.

Reviews research, treatment approaches, and intervention strategies related to problems experienced by children of alcoholics. Research suggests that these children have low self-esteem, are easily frustrated, often perform poorly in school, are at high risk of developing alcoholism, and are more likely than their peers to develop other adjustment problems. It is suggested that early intervention programs must use aggressive outreach to locate and assist children of alcoholics, the entire family can benefit from treatment when one or both parents are alcoholic and existing services need to be expanded.

557. Hirsch, R. (1975). A family therapy approach to the treatment of drug abuse and addiction. Journal of psychedelic drugs, 7(2), 181-185.

Suggests ways of using the family dynamics of the addict as a tool for evaluating and working with addicts and their families. The study examines 47 families of drug abusers. Many of these had multigenerational histories of excessive alcohol use as a coping device and of the utilization of psychotropic drugs to decrease parental anxiety.

558. Howe, B. (1974). Family therapy and the treatment of drug abuse problems. Family therapy, 1(1), 89-98.

Describes the potential role for the family therapist in drug abuse treatment. The question of who is actually having a problem in cases of youthful drug abuse is considered, and the general rule that "the crazier your patient acts, the more likely it is that he is being accurate" is proposed. Drug abuse is seen as a way to dissipate anxiety in a family or social system. When the anxiety reaches a tolerable level for everyone in the system, the cues for delinquent behavior will disappear and the behavior will abruptly cease.

559. Janzen, C. (1977). Families in the treatment of alcoholism. Journal of studies on alcohol, 38(1), 114-130.

Reviews the literature available on family treatment of alcoholism and suggests that, although there is neither a single definition of family therapy nor a single theory behind it, there is agreement that family therapy can be beneficial for both the alcoholic and the family. Most of the reported family treatment was concurrent with or subsequent to other treatment.

560. Janzen, C. (1978). Family treatment for alcoholism: A review. Social work, 23(2), 135-141.

Reviews the social work literature in an attempt to clarify the nature of the relationship between the problems of the family and the problem of the alcoholic. The author emphasizes that families of alcoholics are transacting systems, and concludes with a brief review of several treatment programs.

561. Kaufman, E., and Kaufman, P. (1977). Multiple family therapy: A new direction in the treatment of drug abusers. American journal of drug and alcohol abuse, 4(4), 467-478.

Presents multiple family therapy as an important treatment augmentation for drug abusers in a variety of settings. The total family is viewed as the patient, with the drug abuser as the symptom bearer.

562. Kern, J., and others. (1977). A treatment approach for children of alcoholics. Journal of drug education, 7(3), 207-217.

Describes the need for treatment programs to focus on the needs of children who have alcoholic parents to prevent the development of a second generation of alcoholics. This paper describes the efforts of an education, prevention program for children and their mothers to address this issue. Recommendations for future programming are offered.

563. McKamy, L. (1976). Multiple Family Therapy on an alcohol treatment unit. Family therapy, 3(3), 197-209.

Reports on the usage of multiple family therapy on an alcoholism unit. Cites examples of successful therapeutic techniques in areas such as support, confrontation, interpretation, and improvement in family communication. Family communication is seen as a key ingredient in the development of alcoholism and, therefore, a key to successful prevention efforts.

564. Milner, G. (1977). The treatment of alcoholic and drug dependent persons in Victoria. *Journal of drug issues*, *7*(4), 385-389.

Summarized the development of a multidisciplinary, community-oriented treatment, research, and rehabilitation program for alcoholics and drug abusers. May be used as a secondary prevention model for youthful substance abusers.

565. O'Connor, W., and Morgan, D. (1968). Multidisciplinary treatment of alcoholism: A consultation program for team coordination. *Quarterly journal of studies on alcohol*, *29*(4-A), 903-908.

Describes the interdisciplinary approach to the treatment of alcoholics and their families and a community consultation program.

566. Rueveni, U., and Wiener, M. (1976). Network intervention of disturbed families: The key role of network activists. *Psychotherapy: Theory, research and practice*, *13*(2), 173-176.

Descibes the development of a network approach to treatment for a family. Such treatment may be helpful as a prevention and treatment approach for drug and alcohol abusing families.

567. Shapiro, R. (1977). A family therapy approach to alcoholism. *Journal of marriage and family counseling*, *3*(4), 71-78.

Presents data from recent studies that strongly suggest that family therapy is a promising method of treatment for alcoholism. A comprehensive treatment program is presented.

568. Solow, R., and Cooper, B. (1974). Therapeutic mobilization of families around drug induced adolescent crises. Adolescent psychiatry, 3, 237-248.

Discusses the crises induced in families by drug-abusing adolescents. Drug abuse is described as the drug user's attempt to effect individuation.

569. Steinglass, P. (1976). Experimenting with family treatment approaches to alcoholism, 1950-1975: A review. Family process, 15(1), 97-123.

Presents a critical review of experimental and clinical studies conducted over the last 25 years on the use of family therapy in the treatment of alcoholism. The author offers possible explanations for the reluctance of family therapists to treat this problem more effectively.

* Wunderlich, R., Lozes, J., and Lewis, J. (1974). Recidivism rates of group therapy participants and other adolescents processed by a juvenile court. Psychotherapy: Therapy, research, and practice, 11(3), 243-245.

See No. 373.

Role of Parents

570. Allen, T. (1984). Teens and drugs: Everyone's business. Focus on family and chemical dependency, 7(1), 10-11.

Discusses the ways that parents, schools, and communities deny the existence of alcohol and drug problems. The author describes ways to help break through this denial and the responsibilities each must take on. Recommendations for prevention programs are included.

* Babst, D., Miran, M., and Koval, M. (1976). The relationship between friends' marijuana use, family cohesion, school interest, and drug abuse prevention. Journal of drug education, 6(1), 23-41.

See No. 418.

571. Bry, B. (1983). Empirical foundations of family-based approaches to adolescent substance abuse. In: Preventing adolescent drug abuse: Intervention strategies. Rockville, MD: National Institute on Drug Abuse.

Presents a discussion of family-based prevention approaches. A description of the etiology of drug abuse, including the role the family plays in this, is given. Evidence is presented to support family involvement and how it can reduce substance abuse precursors and early signs of abuse.

572. Eiseman, S. (1974). An approach to primary prevention of drug abuse among children and youth--parental influence. Journal of drug education, 4(1), 27-35.

Offers guidelines for effective parent-child relationships. Describes these guidelines as one way parents can have a positive influence on child development.

* Forrest, G. (1983). How to cope with a teenage drinker: New alternatives and hope for parents and families. New York, NY: Atheneum.

See No. 384.

573. Garfield, E., and Gibbs, J. (1982). Fostering parent involvement for drug prevention. Journal of drug education, 12(2), 87-96.

Describes the needs of parents to support each other through mutual support groups. Further, describes the formation of such groups with suggested consideration for start-up and continuation ideas.

574. Gluckstern, N. (1973). Training parents as drug counselors in the community. Personnel and guidance journal, 51, 676-680.

Describes a program designed to educate parents with regard to drugs, to train them in counseling and human relations, and to support them with follow-up services as they enter the community.

575. Huberty, C., and Huberty, D. (1976). Treating the parents of adolescent drug abusers. Contemporary drug problems, 5(4), 573-592.

Outlines a program for the rehabilitation of parents of drug-abusing youth. Describes these families as suffering due to a variety of stated reasons all related to the members' drug abuse. Didactic methods which lead to more affective communications are described.

576. Jacobson, M. (1983, January). Parent movement in the United States. Paper presented at the Tenth Biennial Summer School of the National Society on Alcoholism and Drug Dependency, Wellington, New Zealand.

Discusses and lists various stages parents may find themselves in regarding their child's drug usage. This list is compiled to be concurrent to the various stages of treatment. A list of signs and symptoms are presented as well as an outline for a neighborhood plan for prevention of drug abuse.

577. Kearney, A. (1979). Drug abuse and your child: What can the schools do? School counselor, 26(3), 187-190.

Describes a prevention program that has as its premise that drug abuse is a people problem and that people who use drugs have problems, and that drug abuse is just a symptom of these problems.

* Kern, J., and others. (1977). A treatment approach for children of alcoholics. Journal of drug education, 7(3), 207-217.

See No. 562.

* Kinard, B. (1982). 97th Congress, February 1982, Testimony of Beverly J. Kinard. In: Hearing ... Ninety-Seventh Congress. Salt Lake City, UT: Utah Congress of Parents and Teachers.

See No. 255.

* Koberl, I. (1981). Thoughts on drug prevention and prophylaxis. Weiner zeitschrift fuer such Forschung, 4(1), 17-19.

See No. 260.

* Kruger, W.S. (1972). Education for parenthood and the schools. Washington, DC: Bureau of Elementary and Secondary Education.

See No. 11.

* Lassey, M., and Carlson, J. (1981). Teenage drinking in Idaho's rural communities. Moscow, ID: University of Idaho College of Agriculture.

See No. 110.

* Lipton, W. (1977, June). Alcohol handicapped child. Paper presented at the 23rd International Institute on Prevention and Treatment of Alcoholism, Dresden, Germany.

See No. 269.

* McDonald, D. (1982). Progressive stages of teenage drug abuse. In: PRIDE Southeast Drug Conference Proceedings 1980 and 1981. Atlanta, GA: PRIDE.

See No. 391.

578. Mental Health Materials Center. (1979). A selective guide to audiovisuals for mental health and family life education. Chicago, IL: Marquis Academic Media.

Contains references to audiovisual materials on alcohol and drug abuse. Also included: halfway houses, suicide and crisis intervention, delinquency, adolescent mental health, child abuse, and developmental disabilities. There are some chapters devoted to how to effectively use print and audiovisual materials.

579. Mental Health Materials Center. (1979). A selective guide to audiovisuals for mental health and family life education. Chicago, IL: Marquis Academic Media.

Its 949 pages are devoted to aspects of drug abuse prevention and mental health. Particularly useful for therapeutic communities and prevention programs where the mental health of the clients is the key to a drug-free life.

* National Institute on Alcohol Abuse and Alcoholism. (1984). Prevention plus: Involving schools, parents, and the community in alcohol and drug education. Rockville, MD: Author.

See No. 13.

* National Institute of Drug Abuse. (1980). Angel dust in four American cities: An ethnographic study of PCP users. Kensington, MD: Author.

See No. 602.

* National Institute of Drug Abuse. (1980). For kids only: What you should know about marijuana. (DHHS Pub. No. 80-986). Rockville, MD: Author.

See No. 604.

580. National Institute on Drug Abuse. (1980). For Parents only: What you need to know about marijuana. Rockville, MD: Author.

Companion guide to For Kids only: What you should know about marijuana. Assists parents in working with their children in the development of knowledge about marijuana abuse and prevention. Includes drug abuse identification information. See No. 604 for information about the primary text.

* PTA Today. (1982). How you can help your child make responsible decisions about drinking. PTA Today, 7(4), 6-b.

See No. 395.

581. Public Affairs Committee. (1980). Children and drugs. New York: Author.

Contains advice for parents, a brief description of effects of various drugs, and signs of possible drug use to watch for in children. Appears to make no revolutionary new statements in the field, but may be useful as a brief overview with useful statistics.

* Rehrer, R. (1982). Now what do I do? A guide on alcohol and drugs for youth. St. Louis, MO: Concordia Publishing House.

See No. 399.

582. Reinhart, R. (1974). The family drug awareness group: A citizen initiated example for effective community concern. Journal of drug education, 4(2), 151-155.

Describes and explores a model of prevention education that has been adopted in an area in southern California where there was a high incidence of drug abuse. The project was built on parental involvement and the authors suggest that this project may have applicability for other regions.

* Schuchard, M. (1982). National parents' movement for drug-free youth. In: PRIDE Southeast Drug Conference Proceedings, 1980 and 1981. Atlanta, GA: PRIDE.

See No. 326.

* Smith, E. (1981). Adolescent drug abuse and alcoholism: Directions for the school and the family. Urban education, 16(3), 311-322.

See No. 336.

* Spazzapan, B., and DeVanna, M. (1981). Cultural aspects of alcoholic habits in lower middle schools. Minerva psichiatrica, 22(4), 177-182.

See No. 407.

* Stepien, H. (1979). Preventive action among children and adolescents. Problemy Alkoholizmu, 26(3), 4-8.

See No. 340.

583. Twerski, A. (1981). Caution: Kindness can be dangerous to the alcoholic. Englewood Cliffs, NJ: Prentice hall.

Deals with identification of alcoholism, parent-child and child-parent relationships, on the job situations, drinking and driving, doctor-patient relationships, confrontations, and ineffective home remedies.

* United States Jaycees. (1975). All in the family: Understanding how we teach and influence children about alcohol. Participants' workbook and chairman's guide. Tulsa, OK: Author.

See No. 490.

* Vejnoska, J. (1982). Parent action groups: A prevention resource. Alcohol health and research world, 6(4), 13-17.

See No. 362.

584. Woodward, N. (1981). If your child is drinking ... What you can do to fight alcohol abuse at home, at school, and in the community. New York: G.P. Putnam's Sons.

Offers advice to parents on how to deal with children and alcohol. Provides a program outline for children who drink while offering support for their parents. Emphasis is given to the importance of viewing and treating a child's alcohol problem as one that affects the entire family.

* Wunderlich, R., Lozes, J., and Lewis, J. (1974). Recidivism rates of group therapy participants and other adolescents processed by a juvenile court. Psychotherapy: Therapy, research, and practice, 11(3), 243-245.

See No. 373.

PUBLICATIONS

585. Addiction Research Foundation. (1981). Core knowledge in the drug field. Ontario, Canada: Author.

Presents a twelve-part set of writings on the many aspects of drug abuse treatment, education, prevention, economics, etiology, history, pharmacology, and other areas of drug abuse.

586. American Association for Health, Physical Education, and Recreation. (1969). Research book for drug abuse information. Washington, DC: National Science Teachers Association.

Presents materials about teaching about drugs, facts about drugs, and supplemental reports that deal with prevention, drug use, and student value correlates, motivation, etc. The section that deals with teaching about drugs presents practical and concrete suggestions for elementary and secondary school teachers, as well as administrators. Much of the focus is built around communication with youth.

587. American Association for Marriage and Family Therapy, AMFT newsletter. Upland, CA.

Written for professionals in marital and family therapy. Interesting for readers who deal with families that are enmeshed in alcohol and drug concerns as a symptom of other underlying problems.

588. Balster, R., and Ellinwood, E. (1974). Resource materials for drug abuse professionals: An individualized reading list.

Journal of drug education, 4(3), 295-299.

Describes the Duke University Drug Abuse Reference Project (DUDARP). This is a system for personalizing a list of resource materials for professionals in the area of drug abuse treatment and prevention.

* Bayh, B. (1975). Our nation's schools--A report card: "A" in school violence and vandalism. Preliminary report of the Subcommittee to investigate juvenile delinquency. Washington, DC: Congress of the U.S., Senate Committee on the Judiciary.

See No. 156.

* Braucht, G. (1982). Problem drinking among adolescents: A review and analysis of psychosocial research. In: Alcohol and health monograph No. 4: Special population issues. Washington, DC: U.S. Government Printing Office.

See No. 377.

589. Center for Alcohol Studies. (1980). Recent Topics in Alcohol Studies. Piscataway, NJ: Rutgers University.

Compiled by the Alcohol Information Retrieval System (AIRS). Contains a data base of computer-generated bibliographies with abstracts providing overviews of the recent international scientific/technical literature on over 60 subject areas. The multidisciplinary material offers information for researchers, clinicians, educators, or administrators seeking information on a wide range of alcohol related subjects.

590. The Center for Youth Development and Research. (1980). The youthwork bibliography. St. Paul, MN: Author.

Covers 16 major sections including drugs, health, sexuality, deviance, and youth participation. Includes descriptions of newsletters, journals, films, and sources. Developed by the National Youthworker Education Project, it covers the years 1975-1980.

591. Erickson, P. (1980). Cannabis Criminals. Addiction Research Foundation: Ontario, Canada.

Presents various aspects of law and social policy regarding drug abuse in general. Of use to those interested in prevention as it relates to the connections between criminal justice and drug using behavior.

592. Essence of adolescence. Highland Park, NJ: Essence Publications.

A newsletter, published 11 times yearly, on problems of youth and those who help--parents, teachers, administrators in various agencies. Issues generally contain information pertaining to alcohol and drug problems, mental health, primary prevention topics, parenting, and much more.

593. Gone Way Down. (1983). St. Petersburg, FL: Straight, Inc.

Presents a lecture by Miller Newton, the medical director of Straight, Inc. The lecture describes drug abuse as a "disease of the feelings" in which drug use forms the central problem, as a chronic, progressive, and terminal disease.

* Harford, T., and Spiegler, D. (1982). Environmental influences in adolescent drinking. In: Alcohol and health monograph No. 4: Special populations. Washington, DC: U.S. Government Printing Office.

See No. 385.

594. Heath, D., and Cooper, A. (1981). Alcohol use and world cultures: A comprehensive bibliography of anthropological sources. Ontario, Canada: Addictions Research Foundation.

Presents part of an extensive bibliographic series which began in 1968. The citations are not annotated, therefore, it can only be used as a guide for other research.

* Hewitt, L. (1982). Current status of alcohol education programs for youth. In: Alcohol and health mono. no. 4: Special populations. Washington, DC: U.S. Government Printing Office.

See No. 102.

595. Journal of Psychoactive Drugs, San Francisco, CA.

Published originally as The Journal of Psychadelic Drugs, its name was changed to reflect more current concerns. It maintains a focus on the treatment and prevention of drug and alcohol abuse.

596. Kopita, R. (1973). Searchlight: Relevant resources in high interest areas. 4U update search. Counseling for drug abuse. Ann Arbor, MI: ERIC Clearinghouse on Counseling and Personnel Services.

Reviews 70 document abstracts retrieved from the ERIC collection, Dissertation Abstracts, and the journal literature, and covers techniques and school programs for education and prevention of drug abuse.

597. McEwen, W., and Hannenman, G. (1972, December). Public service advertising and social problems: The case of drug abuse prevention. Paper presented at the Annual Meeting of the Speech Communication Association, Chicago, IL.

Explores certain findings of a DAIR (Drug Abuse Information Research) project undertaken at the University of Connecticut which investigated the dissemination and impact of drug abuse information.

598. Mental Health Materials Center. (1979). A

selective guide to publications for mental health and family life education. Chicago, IL: Marquis Academic Media.

Presents many aspects of the mental health field that interrelate with drug and alcohol abuse and further suggests prevention strategies for all.

* Messolonghites, L. (1976). Primary prevention in drug abuse: An annotated guide to the literature. Rockville, MD: National Institute on Drug Abuse.

See No. 279.

599. Milgram, G. (1978). Alcohol education materials 1973-1978: An annotated bibliography. New Brunswick, NJ: Rutgers Center of Alcohol Studies.

Lists 686 publications issued over a 6-year period by almost every publisher and nonprofit organization that makes their materials available to the public. Contains 100 titles which indicates that a least 15-20% are out of date. The focus is primarily on alcohol and includes a great many drug publications that have relevance to alcohol use and prevention.

600. MTI Teleprograms, Inc. (1979). Joy's Story, Schiller Park, IL: Author.

Talks about the consequences of using drugs. After undergoing hospital treatment for five months, a 13-year-old girl describes her experiences using drugs. It is an incomplete story, and is of doubtful use as a prevention tool in the classroom, a teaching aid for counselors or teachers since it offers no apparent solution or suggestions that have practical application.

601. National Clearinghouse for Alcohol Information. (1976). Selected publications on education and training about alcohol. Report Number: DHEW-ADW-76-272. Rockville, MD: Author.

Describes the Grouped Interest Guides that are produced by the Acquisition and Reference Services of the National Clearinghouse for Alcohol Information, an information service of the National Institute on Alcohol Abuse and Alcoholism. The aim is to provide the reader with a regularly published series of bibliographic references for recent, topical literature in the designated areas. This guide is a cumulative issue of previously published editions.

602. National Institute of Drug Abuse. (1980). Angel dust in four American cities: An ethnographic study of PCP users. Kensington, MD: Author.

Covers the cities of Miami, Seattle, Philadelphia, and Chicago. Highly recommended reading for anyone dealing with PCP users; which the authors indicate is probably 90% of youth service agencies in the United States. Single copies free.

603. National Institute of Drug Abuse. (1981). Catalogue of Services Research Reports/Monographs/Manuals. Kensington, MD: Author.

Contains 65 different publications with 25 major subject headings. This 20-page catalogue of technical publications is available free on a single copy basis.

604. National Institute of Drug Abuse. (1980). For kids only: What you should know about marijuana. (DHHS Pub. No. 80-986). Rockville, MD: Author.

Contains simple text aimed at pre-teens, using few simple complex words and many short sentences. No mention regarding why young people would want to try this drug, or what some of the more problematic, subjective efforts might be. Contains large type and frequent illustrations which make it easy reading. Single copies are available free. Has a counterpart publication, For parents only: What you need to know about marijuana, see no. 580.

* National Institute of Drug Abuse. (1980). For parents only: What you need to know about marijuana. (DHHS Pub. No. 80-986). Rockville, MD: Author.

See No. 580.

605. National Institute of Mental Health. (1971). A guide to drug abuse education and information materials. Chevy Chase, MD: National Clearinghouse for Drug Abuse Information.

Presents drug abuse materials developed by and available through the National Institute of Mental Health, National Clearinghouse for Drug Abuse Information. The presented materials span many various media including materials relevant and designed for use in the classroom.

606. National Institute of Mental Health. (1971). Drug abuse prevention: A guide to speakers. Chevy Chase, MD: National Clearinghouse for Drug Abuse Information.

Designed as a resource for persons requiring knowledge about speaker's bureaus concerned with drug abuse prevention throughout the country. No attempt at evaluation is made.

607. National Institute of Mental Health. Drug dependence and abuse: A selected bibliography. (1971). Chevy Chase, MD: National Clearinghouse for Drug Abuse Information.

Presented a selected list of references designed to provide an introduction to both scientific and popular drug abuse literature. This bibliography specifies 21 major subject areas developed through working with the literature and consulting experts.

608. Nellis, M., (Ed.). (1972). Resource book on drug abuse education, (3rd Ed.). Rockville, MD: NIDA.

Presents a collection of materials on the scientific, philosophical, and educational aspects of drug abuse literature. This publication serves as a basis for improved understanding, trust, and communication between teacher and student concerning drug use.

609. Nowlis, H. (1980, March). Prevention is not easy. Paper presented at the First Pan-Pacific Conference on Drugs and Alcohol, Canberra, Australia.

Discusses the distinctions between information and education, and between these teaching methods and prevention. Definitions of prevention are suggested. The author concludes that the field should move away from focusing on pharmacological issues and move towards a multidimensional social behavior model.

610. Nowlis, H. (1977). Statement before the Subcommittee on Alcoholism and Drug Abuse, Committee on Human Resources, United States Senate. Washington, DC: United States Government Printing Office.

Presents the Drug Education Program funded by the Education Personnel Development funds of the Office of Education. After establishing several projects, the team leaders felt their most valuable role would be one of leadership, training, and resources, through a network of regional resource centers. Training is offered and includes needs assessments; program planning; team building; group, individual, and peer counseling. No evaluation data is presented.

* Schluetter, W. (1980). Alcohol, drugs or alternatives: A film discussion guide. Minneapolis, MN: University of Minnesota, Continuing Education in Social Work.

See No. 325.

* Strategy Council on Drug Abuse, Washington, D.C. (1974). Federal strategy for drug abuse and drug traffic prevention. Washington, DC: United States Government Printing Office.

See No. 341.

* Swiss Institute for Alcoholism Prevention. (1982). Newsletter. October 29, 1982. Lausanne, Switzerland: Author.

See No. 349.

611. The White House Conference for a Drug Free America, Final Report. (1988, June). Washington, DC: United States Government Printing Office.

Presents the findings of a conference, hosted by the White House, on all aspects related to substance abuse and alcohol abuse in America. Includes specific recommendations on prevention as it relates to educational services and programs as well as sources of information on and resources for substance abuse.

APPENDIX 1

Sources of Information and Resources

In addition to the literature reviews in the previous chapters, the following associations, publishers, agencies, and service providers are sources of information, literature, and other materials, as well as being available for further research. These will be helpful to anyone wishing to obtain further information on services, materials, literature, program development, funding, etc.

ACTION
Drug Prevention Program
806 Connecticut Ave., N.W.
Washington, DC 20525

The Action Drug Alliance's goal is to strengthen and expand community-based drug abuse prevention. Their services include the development of programs, grants, conferences, and other forms of technical assistance.

Adult Children of Alcoholics
Central Service Board
P.O. Box 3216
Torrence, CA 90505

This is a central clearinghouse for those interested in the development of programs that specialize in serving the needs of children of alcoholics. This is based on the 12-step tradition of A.A. The groups were originally designed to meet the needs of the adult children of alcoholics but have recently begun to identify and meet the needs of children.

Al-Anon Family Group Headquarters
P.O. Box 862
Midtown Station
New York, NY 10018-0862

This is the central headquarters and clearinghouse for the national association for Al-Anon, the family program for alcoholics and members of A.A.

Alcoholics Anonymous
Box 459
Grand Central Station
New York, NY 10163

This is the central headquarters for the international fellowship of Alcoholics Anonymous. They offer referral services, literature, and other sources of information of alcohol abuse, prevention, and A.A. meetings.

American Bar Association
Advisory Commission on Youth, Alcohol, and Drug Problems
A.B.A.
1800 M Street, N.W.
Washington, DC 20036

American Council for Drug Education (ACDE)
Suite 110
204 Monroe Street
Rockville, MD 20850

The ACDE is an organization which specializes in the development of educational materials, reviews of scientific findings, as well as developing educational media campaigns. Most of their materials are targeted towards educational personnel, parents, physicians, and other human service employees.

The American Legion
A Square Deal for Every Child
National Americanism and Children and Youth Division
P.O. Box 1055
Indianapolis, IN 46206

This service makes literature available as well as speakers who will address groups of students on the facts about drug and alcohol abuse.

American Prosecutors Research Institute
Center for Local Prosecution of Drug Offenses
1033 North Fairfax Street
Suite 200
Alexandria, VA 22314

This agency arranges for training, technical assistance, and effective techniques in dealing with drug abuse cases to local prosecutors.

Benevolent and Protective Order of Elks
Drug Awareness Program
P.O. Box 310
Ashland, OR 97520

This group distributes literature on substance abuse to local schools and other community-based organizations. Speakers on the subject of alcohol and drug abuse prevention are available.

Cocanon Family Groups
P.O. Box 64742-66
Los Angeles, CA 90064

This is a listing of services for the family members of cocaine abusers.

Comp Care Publications
2415 Annapolia Lane
Minneapolis, MN 55441

Comp Care Publications is a source of pamphlets, books, charts and other materials on drug abuse, prevention, and self-help programs.

Drug Enforcement Administration
1405 Eye Street, N.W.
Washington, DC 20537

The D.E.A. offers a wide variety of information on the development of treatment and prevention programs. Literature, films, and other materials are also available. This office has, at times, funded demonstration grants for the purpose of prevention and treatment.

Families Anonymous
P.O. Box 528
Van Nuys, CA 91408

This is a self-help program based on the 12-step traditions of A.A. for the families and friends of drug abusers.

Hazeldon Educational Materials
Box 176
Center City, MN 55012

Hazeldon publishes a wide variety of materials related to both alcohol and drug abuse. Materials are available in all medias. Materials are suitable for prevention, treatment, and in recovery programs. The needs of all family members are addressed.

Kiwanis International
Public Relations
3636 Woodview Terrace
Indianapolis, IN 46268

Materials and information related to the public awareness of drug and alcohol abuse are available. These are generally geared towards use for billboards, radio, T.V., and public service announcements. They have also developed a teaching manual, for grades 4 through 6, entitled: Choices about drugs.

Lions Club International
Special Research and Development
300 22nd Street
Oakbrook, IL 60570

The staff of the Lions Club have developed drug awareness materials that emphasize drug abuse prevention. This is done primarily through education and includes information on how to get involved in community activities. In conjunction with Quest International, the Lions have developed a curriculum entitled: Skills for adolescents. This is geared towards youth, 10-14 years of age, and teaches them to make responsible decisions and how to contend with negative peer pressure.

Mothers Against Drunk Drivers (MADD)
National Office
669 Airport Freeway, Suite 310
Hurst, TX 76053

MADD sponsors public awareness campaigns against drinking while driving. They actively pursue the development of public policies, legislation, and programs geared towards the development of non-drunk driving.

Nar-Anon Family Group Headquarters
World Service Headquarters
P.O. Box 2562
Palos Verdes Peninsula, CA 90274

This is the family support group for members of Narcotics Anonymous and others suffering from drug abuse. It is based on the 12-step traditions of A.A. and is open to friends of drug abusers.

Narcotics Anonymous
World Service Office
P.O. Box 9999
Van Nuys, CA 91409

This is a group program developed on the philosophy of A.A. and offers support to drug abusers in a self-help fashion. N.A. has 12,000 chapters in the United States and chapters in 40 other countries.

Narcotics Education, Inc.
6830 Laurel Street, N.W.
Washington, DC 20012

Publishes literature, books, teaching aids, posters, audio-visuals, and magazines with drug-free messages.

National Association for
Children of Alcoholics (NACOA)
31582 Coast Highway, Suite B
South Laguna, CA 92677

NACOA publishes magazines, pamphlets, and other information for children of alcoholics. Information on meetings are arranged through the A.C.A., listed above.

National Association of
Juvenile and Family Court Judges
P.O. Box 8970
University of Nevada/Reno
Judicial College Building, #18
Reno, NV 89507

This association provides a report, Juvenile and family substance abuse: A judicial response. In addition, it provides technical assistance on issues of dependency, delinquency, and general substance abuse problems. Information on screening, assessment, prevention, and treatment are also available.

National Association of
Secondary School Principals (NASSP)
1904 Association Drive
Reston, VA 22091

The goal of this association is to advance middle and high school education and provides leadership in such matters as administration, supervision, research, professional standards, and educational problems. Can be used as a resource for any secondary school principal.

National Board of YWCA
of the U.S.A.
726 Broadway
New York, NY 10003

The YWCA promotes a combined drug and alcohol prevention program for young girls and women entitled: Women as preventers: An adult-teen partnership.

National Clearinghouse for Alcohol
and Drug Abuse Information (NCADI)
P.O. Box 2345
Rockville, MD 20852

The Clearinghouse operates under the Office of Substance Abuse Prevention and has available an extensive library that covers a range of alcohol and drug abuse, prevention, and treatment issues. The library has a computerized search staff that can trace any relevant topic. Bulk quantities of literature are available to the general public.

National Commission on Resources for Youth (NCRY)
36 West 44th Street
New York, NY 10036

Publishes a quarterly newsletter, Resources for Youth; maintains a library of films, books, guides, and how-to manuals. In addition, the Commission has available descriptions of 1,500 youth participation programs, offers direct assistance to youth programs by acting as an information sharing resource, conducts workshops, and hosts conferences.

National Council on Alcoholism
12 West 21st Street
New York, NY 10010

The National Council's goal is to provide educational and advocacy on behalf of alcoholics, their families, and other drug abusers. There are over 200 affiliate councils throughout the United States representing individual communities.

National Child Safety Council
P.O. Box 1386
Jackson, MI 49204

This group produces booklets, kits, and other materials for educators on drug abuse prevention subjects.

National Diffusion Network (NDN)
Division of Education Replication

U.S. Department of Education
ROB 3, Room 3616
400 Maryland Avenue, S.W.
Washington, DC 20202

This project identifies school-based programs that have been proven effective and can be replicated in other school districts. NDN staff help schools identify their needs and match or develop an educational program to address these needs. Many of these programs are detailed in Educational Programs that Work.

National Institute on Alcoholism
and Alcohol Abuse
U.S. Department of
Health and Human Services
5600 Fishers Lane
Rockville, MD 20857

Provides information on alcoholism and alcoholism prevention for the general public. Has an extensive library on the subject that is available for the public.

National Institute on Drug Abuse (NIDA)
U.S. Department of Health
and Human Services
5600 Fishers Lane
Rockville, MD 20857

Materials, information, technical assistance on the prevention treatment of drug abuse are available. NIDA conducts and sponsors grants for research and services on the causes of, as well as the treatment and prevention of, drug abuse.

National Institute on Health
U.S. Department of Health
and Human Services
9000 Rockville Pike
Bethesda, MD

Offers technical assistance, literature, brochures, and information on preventive health issues. Research grants are available for issues of prevention and treatment.

National Institute on Mental Health
U.S. Department of Health and Human Services
560 Fishers Lane
Rockville, MD 20857

Like the other institutes of the Department of Health and Human Services, research is the primary focus. Literature, brochures, and other types of information are available.

National Organization on Legal Problems of Education
3601 Southwest 29th
Suite 223
Topeka, KS 66614

The National Organization on Legal Problems of Education provides information on the legal aspects of education including those relating to drug use in educational institutions.

National Parent-Teacher Association (P.T.A.)
700 North Rush Street
Chicago, IL 60611-2571

This association provides information on the aspects of communication with children as it relates to drug and alcohol prevention. It is available as a resource for groups wishing to develop prevention programs in schools.

National School Boards Association
Council of School Attorneys
1680 Duke Street
Alexandria, VA 22314

This organization conducts programs and seminars, as well as publishing monographs, on a wide range of topics including drug abuse and the effects this can have on school districts.

National Self-Help Clearinghouse
33 West 42nd Street

Room 620-N
New York, NY 10036

Provides information and training on self-help, carries out research activities, maintains a data bank for self-help referrals, and publishes manuals, training materials, and a newsletter.

Students to Offset Peer
Pressure (S.T.O.P.P.)
10 Lindsey Street
Hudson, NH 03051

Provides information and technical assistance on implementing drug prevention programs.

Toughlove
P.O. Box 1069
Doylestown, PA 18901

Promotes self-help groups for parents, children, and friends of youth who are having problems with drug or alcohol abuse, truancy, or delinquency.

U.S. Department of Education
Drug-Free Schools and Communities
400 Maryland Avenue, S.W.
Washington, DC 20202-4101

Through its five regional centers, technical assistance is offered for the development of programs that lessen the incidents of drug and alcohol abuse. Funding for such projects is also arranged through cooperatively developed state grants.

Washington Legal Foundation
Courtwatch
1705 N Street, N.W.
Washington, DC

Courtwatch is a program that monitors what happens to accused drug dealers in the court system.

Wisconsin Clearinghouse
1954 East Washington Avenue
Madison, WI 53794

This is the official source of information for the State of Wisconsin. It offers a wide variety of publications, materials, agencies available for consultation, in Wisconsin, and in the remaining states.

Youth Who Care
Box 4074
Grand Junction, CO 81502

Provides information on the development of drug abuse prevention programs for youth.

APPENDIX 2

Periodicals available on drug and alcohol abuse

The following list of periodicals is intended for those who wish to pursue further research or obtain linkages for on-going updates in the field. In addition to the journal title, the name and address of the publisher is provided.

Addiction and Substance Report
667 Madison Avenue
New York, NY 10021

Addictions
Addiction Research Foundation of Ontario
33 Russell Street
Toronto, M5S 2S1

Alcohol & Drug Awareness Newsletter
Alcohol & Drug Abuse Division
Department of Social & Rehab. Service
State Office Bldg.
Montpelier, VT 05602

The Alcoholism Report
JSL Reports
1120 National Press Bldg.
Washington, DC 20045

Contemporary Drug Problems
Federal Legal Publs., Inc.
95 Morton Street
New York, NY 10014

Drug Abuse & Alcoholism Review
The Haworth Press
149 Fifth Avenue
New York, NY 10010

<u>Drug Forum--The Journal of Human Issues</u>
Baywood Publ. Co., Inc.
120 Marine Street
Farmingdale, NY 11735

<u>Drug Survival News</u>
Do It Now Foundation
P.O. Box 5115
Phoenix, AR 85010

<u>Focal Points</u>
National Clearinghouse for Smoking and Health
Bureau of Health Education
Public Health Service
Atlanta, GA 30333

<u>Grassroots</u>
Student Assoc. for the Study of Hallucinogens (STASH)
118 South Bedford Street
Madison, WI 53703

<u>International Journal of Altered States</u>
Baywood Publ. Co.
120 Marine Street
Farmingdale, NY 11735

<u>The Journal</u>
Addiction Research Foundation of Ontario
33 Russell Street
Toronto, M5S 2SS1

<u>Journal of Alcohol and Drug Education</u>
The Alcohol and Drug Problems Assoc. of North America (ADPA)
11011 115th Street, N.W.
Suite 204
Washington, DC 20005

<u>Journal of Drug Issues</u>
P.O. Box 4021
Tallahassee, FL 32303

Journal of Psychedelic Drugs
118 South Bedford Street
Madison, WI 53703

Legislative Alerts
National Assoc. of State Drug
Abuse Program Coordinators
1612 K Street, N.W.
Suite 900
Washington, DC 20006

National Coordinating Council
on Drug Education Newsletter
National Drug Reporter
1601 Connecticut Avenue
Washington, DC 20009

National Council on Drug
Abuse Newsletter
Drug/Health Alert
8 South Michigan Avenue
Chicago, IL 60603

NCADI Resources: Update
The National Clearinghouse for
Alcohol and Drug Information
P.O. Box 2345
Rockville, MD 20852

New Mexico Trails
Drug Abuse Division
Dept. of Hospitals and Institutions
113 Washington Avenue
Santa Fe, NM 87501

NIAAA Information & Feature Service
National Institute on Alcohol
Abuse and Alcoholism
5600 Fishers Lane
Rockville, MD 20857

Prevention Pipeline
The National Clearinghouse for
Drug and Alcohol Information
Department PP
P.O. Box 2345
Rockville, MD 20852

Prevention Resources
PYRAMID Project
7101 Wisconsin Avenue
Bethesda, MD 20014

Prevention Update
Center for Multicultural Awareness
2924 Columbia Pike
Arlington, VA 22204

Research Press
2612 North Mattis
Champaign, IL 61820

Rice Paper
Asian-American Drug Abuse Program
5318 Crenshaw Blvd.
Los Angeles, CA 90043

U.S. Journal of Drug and Alcohol Dependance
7541 Biscayne Blvd.
Miami, FL 33138

Washington Drug Review
655 National Press Bldg.
Washington, DC 20045

Wisconsin Association on Alcoholism and Other Drug Abuse, Inc.
Newsletter: WAAODA
333 West Mifflin Street
Madison, WI 53703

AUTHOR INDEX

TITLE INDEX

SUBJECT INDEX